Healthcare Analytics

Foundations and Frontiers

Ross M. Mullner
Edward M. Rafalski

Routledge
Taylor & Francis Group
LONDON AND NEW YORK

Routledge
2 Park Square, Milton Park
Abingdon, Oxon OX14 4RN

Printed on acid-free paper

International Standard Book Number-13: 978-1-4987-5507-8 (Hardback)
978-1-138-19636-0 (Paperback)

Visit the Taylor & Francis Web site at
http://www.taylorandfrancis.com

Contents

Foreword

This is an important book at a critical time in the evolution of our healthcare system. At an average of $8,000 per American, everyone agrees the cost of healthcare is unsustainable, especially for the results we get. It is no wonder that healthcare remains a top priority of government, business, and civic leaders, not to mention ordinary Americans. The rapid development of technology and data have enabled productivity increases to bring down costs in other sectors of the economy, but healthcare has remained stubbornly resistant to these forces. While the policy debate in the media revolves around how to pay for today's healthcare system, many people are working diligently to invent tomorrow's healthcare system—one that costs less, is more patient centered, is easier to access, and is rewarding to practice.

I am one of those people. Ten years ago I left a comfortable job as a partner in a technology investment firm to join all those working toward a better healthcare system. Before leaving for the world of healthcare, I was a self-taught programmer, a management consultant, an entrepreneur and executive at two information technology companies we brought public, and the lead investor in a predictive analytics company that modeled industries and companies using billions of data points and thousands of simultaneous equations. I could see the gap between how data and analytics were revolutionizing other industries, and how elusive that opportunity seemed to be in healthcare. Through my firm AVIA, I now have the opportunity to support dozens of the leading healthcare delivery systems in the United States that are working toward improving the delivery of care by harnessing the power of better technology and troves of data.

Common understanding is that it takes 17 years to move new healthcare evidence into practice. One reason for the delay is the challenge of building up the body of evidence. Every year in the United States, over a million doctors and nurses handle well over a billion visits. We could bring evidence to practice more quickly if we could turn all of those encounters into data, turn the data into insights, and apply the resulting knowledge to the next billion encounters. At the same time, we have the opportunity to revolutionize our knowledge by incorporating literally trillions of pieces of new, more frequent biomarkers. Imagine learning from continuous glucose, heart rate, heart rhythm, respiration, sleep, movement, and stress monitoring data, not to mention the data available from genomics, the microbiome, and the proteome. Finally, what if we could incorporate those insights into designing population-level interventions? Such a system would allow us to shift, dramatically, our focus from treating disease to preventing it. The contribution to reducing costs, improving productivity by delivering the right treatment to the right patient at the right time, and improving the human condition would be enormous. None of this was possible until the cost of a number of technologies to capture, store, and process data came down to their present levels, but now that we are here, we must capture the opportunity.

My experience working with dozens of healthcare systems tells me that we agree broadly about this future, but to usher it into existence will be no mean feat. In *Healthcare Analytics,* Mullner and Rafalski make an important contribution to closing the gap between our vision and our how-to knowledge. We know that data changes everything, but we need a road map for how to architect and use the data, and this book provides it. If you are trying to drive faster data-enabled improvements in the delivery of healthcare, *Healthcare Analytics* is an important read.

Ted Meisel
Co-Founder, AVIA

List of Contributors

James Beem, MHIM, MHA
Managing Director, Global Healthcare Intelligence
J.D. Power
Nashville, Tennessee

Ian M. Brooks, PhD, BSc
Director of Surgical Research
Anne Arundel Medical Center
Annapolis, Maryland

and

Pennsylvania State University
Hyattsville, Maryland

Greg Jordan, PhD, MBA, MA
Founder, Graph Story
University of Memphis
Memphis, Tennessee

Charisse Madlock-Brown, PhD, MA
Assistant Professor
University of Tennessee Health Science Center
Memphis, Tennessee

Razvan Marinescu, MD, MHA, FACHE
Chief Strategy Officer, Memphis Market
Saint Francis Healthcare
Memphis, Tennessee

Ross M. Mullner, PhD
Professor *(retired)*
University of Illinois
School of Public Health
Chicago, Illinois

Pradeep S. B. Podila, PhD, MS, MHA, FACHE, CPHIMS, CPHQ, CHFP, CSSBB
Clinical Research Assistant
Methodist Le Bonheur Healthcare
Memphis, Tennessee

and

PHIFP Fellow at Centers for Disease Control and Prevention
Denver, Colorado

Edward M. Rafalski, PhD, MPH, FACHE
Affiliate Associate Professor
University of South Florida College of Public Health
and
Senior Vice President
Chief Strategy and Marketing Officer
BayCare Health System
Tampa, Florida

Introduction

Healthcare is being disrupted. In a recent McKinsey & Company report, it has been observed that the healthcare industry is going through tectonic shifts that are occurring not only in regulations but in three other areas: technology (both medical science and technology and the onward march of big data, advanced analytics, machine learning, and digital), industry orientation (the move toward business-to-consumer [B2C] and rapidly rising consumer expectations), and reallocation of risk across the value chain. These forces are fundamentally altering the structure of the industry and basis of competition.[1]

The former two shifts, technology and industry orientation, are the drivers of the need to reorient the way in which the healthcare industry must approach analytics into the future. The ubiquitous access to data, both clinical and consumer, affords the healthcare analyst the opportunity to gain insights that can significantly increase value and improve the health of the population, if leveraged appropriately. The former opportunity is estimated to be over $500 billion within the $3 trillion U.S. healthcare economy. This provides significant opportunity for value creation, according to the McKinsey report.[2]

The latter opportunity for improvement is in the reduction of the incidence rates in preventable disease states, such as obesity, that lead to the onset of more complicated health outcomes, such as type II diabetes and cardiovascular disease, which are more expensive to treat. This effort is commonly referred to as population health management. Population health may be defined as the identification of a population and the responsibility for both the health and healthcare of the population. To achieve this, one must focus not only on the healthcare delivery model, but also on the health and well-being of the population. This requires a focus on wellness, preventive care, and control of chronic diseases.[3]

If we are to address the disruptive forces in healthcare directly with analytical solutions, certain foundational skill sets and functions are crucial, such as epidemiological, geospatial, and statistical, central to creating the knowledge necessary to understand utilization patterns and opportunities for improvement.[4] The new frontier in healthcare analytics is the opportunity to harness big data—extremely large consumer data sets that may be analyzed to reveal patterns, trends, and associations, especially relating to human behavior and interactions. The addition of this information can begin to lay the groundwork for linking social determinants of health and health outcomes in near real-time fashion to create value and improve outcomes. Harnessing these massive amounts of data requires a data architecture approach and application of knowledge management. The chapters that follow address the foundational and frontier skills needed to prepare the healthcare industry for its own disruption.

References

1. Singhal S, Latko B, Pardo-Martin, C. *The Future of healthcare: Finding the opportunities that lie beneath the uncertainty.* McKinsey & Company. January, 2018.
2. Ibid.
3. Mayzell, G. Population Health: An Implementation Guide to Improve Outcomes and Lower Costs. Boca Raton: CRC Press; 2016.
4. Ibid.

Chapter 1

Managerial epidemiology: Creating care of health ecosystems

Edward M. Rafalski

CONTENTS

Introduction

Managerial epidemiology combines the science of epidemiology with management principles applied to the improvement of systems of health, whether real or virtual.[1] In this chapter, we explore the future of healthcare analytics from the perspective of studying disease using more recently available data sources to prepare healthcare systems, their analysts, and leaders to create more value for society and the individual consumer.

What is epidemiology?

Epidemiology is the study of how disease is distributed in populations and the factors that influence or determine this distribution.[2] This definition assumes that disease is not random and that characteristics protect or predispose us to disease. It is also the study of the distribution and determinants of health-related states or events in specified populations and the application of this study to the control of health problems.[3] It may also be the study of the distribution and determinants of health and disease in populations, including injuries, accidents, and violence, and the application of this study to promotion of health, prevention of disease, treatment of disease, planning for health and disease, and health policy.[4] Distribution of disease refers to the who, when, and where of an outbreak. Determinants are characteristics that influence whether or not disease occurs. States and events refer to diseases, episodes, and disasters. Disease that affects the population affects a group, not just a single individual.

Regardless of which definition of epidemiology one prefers, the goal is for organizations to be better prepared to deal with future health events and to influence as many variables among target populations as possible to prevent or defer the onset of disease. It is a purpose of public health science and varies, most notably, from medical science given its focus on treating a population versus an individual.

What is managerial epidemiology?

Having a general understanding of epidemiology, the addition of the word "managerial" suggests the application of the principles and tools of epidemiology to the decision-making process in healthcare management. Just as in managerial accounting where the manager is using financial indicators to inform decision-making, the healthcare manager is gleaning information from epidemiological data to inform decision-making.

Integrating epidemiology and its methods into management approaches can be achieved through a number of organizational positions and roles. For example, in strategic planning, the planning analyst is typically looking into the future (usually in the 3- to 5-year horizon) and making recommendations to the organization regarding a suggested course of action based on the best information available on demographics, competitive and regulatory forces, and disease incidence in a target market or population. In staffing and organizing, the human resources analyst is considering how the incidence of disease may influence the need for additional resources. In finance, the analyst is considering the scale of resources required to meet the need or demand for services based on changes in disease incidence in order to calculate a financial return on the investment made. In marketing, the analyst is considering how to motivate the consumer from a precontemplative to a contemplative state and ultimately to act on his or her own health, in other words, to make a healthcare purchase in advance of developing the disease or in the course of managing a chronic condition. In each case, epidemiological data serves as the reference point for informed organizational decision-making.

What is an ecosystem of care?

When thinking about the prevention of disease, segregating the effort into primary, secondary, and tertiary prevention is useful. Primary prevention is focused on avoiding disease altogether, generally by preventing disease development.[5] Weight management/obesity prevention as a precursor to onset of chronic disease, such as hypertension and type II diabetes, is an example. Secondary and tertiary prevention are primarily focused on addressing an illness once it has manifested.

In the primary prevention effort to prevent the onset of obesity, appropriate amounts of diet and exercise can contribute to a successful prevention strategy. When considering how a traditional healthcare system approaches this prevention strategy, assets that are owned or controlled are typically positioned to intervene with the patient in an effort to change behavior. Processes are tested using reliable methodologies, such as Lean/Six Sigma,[6] to standardize workflows, eliminate waste, and achieve consistent outcomes. An example of this approach may include core elements such as primary care, coaching, fitness, nutrition, and mindset/behavioral health (Figure 1.1). Data is captured at each nodal point and integrated into a data warehouse/repository structure enabling the analyst to query the data set to determine outcomes in target populations.[7,8] This is a common model in many health systems across the United States with various flavors and permutations. Some call this *population health* or *accountable care*.

However, the model may have a flaw—healthcare consumers spend more time outside of the healthcare system, on average, than inside of it, thereby limiting the potential for high engagement and meaningful behavioral change. To place the problem in context, consider the following. The average healthcare consumer has an encounter with a health system/provider two to three times per year (within Medicare, the national insurance program for the elderly and disabled, consumers may have four to five encounters). The average grocery shopper may be in the store one to two times per week. Nearly one in five Amazon shoppers are on the site every day making purchases or contemplating purchases.[9]

Consider the primary care annual physical encounter, which typically is an event lasting 15 minutes or less, as an opportunity to generate patient engagement. In that small window of time, a patient at risk for hypertension is encouraged to change behavior, prior to being prescribed a drug(s), depending on where the patient lies on the "disease spectrum." Family history/genetic markers of the disease may lead the physician to be more aggressive in recommending a course of treatment. The patients' spectrum position may lead to the application of additional resources to help the patient reach a goal set by the physician. In accountable care organizations or vertically integrated health systems with a health plan, resources the physician

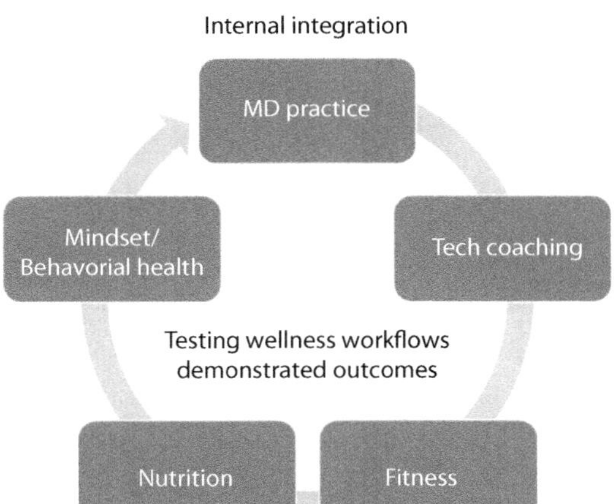

Figure 1.1 Ecosystem of care.

may call on include case/care management. Care management is a set of activities intended to improve patient care and reduce the need for medical services by helping patients and caregivers more effectively manage health conditions. Case management is the coordination of services on behalf of an individual. Unfortunately, case/care management resources are typically reserved for the more chronically ill, qualifying the effort as secondary prevention. What can be done to move the effort to primary prevention?

Case for primary prevention and care of health ecosystem

It has been well established that Americans consume a majority of medical resources in the last 2 years of life.[10] Arguably, our national resources can be better spent earlier in life to prevent unnecessary expenditures at the end of life and thereby lead to a higher quality of life.[11] Unlike healthcare systems with the modern hospital at the center, focused on mostly tertiary prevention, systems of health are organized around and focused on primary prevention. It is a process by which systems are constructed and organized to prevent disease. The intent is to organize resources to more directly address the underlying causes of disease, including lifestyle behaviors, the physical environment, and the social and economic factors influencing health, all of which are generally considered to be outside the realm of (traditional) healthcare. These are generally referred to as the social determinants of health, which explain well over half, or 60%, of health outcomes.[5] Creating an ecosystem of care outside of the four walls of the modern hospital requires a purposeful architecture, beginning with data and program design (Figure 1.2). Consider three use cases to depict how to construct a data-driven care of health ecosystem model for the future.

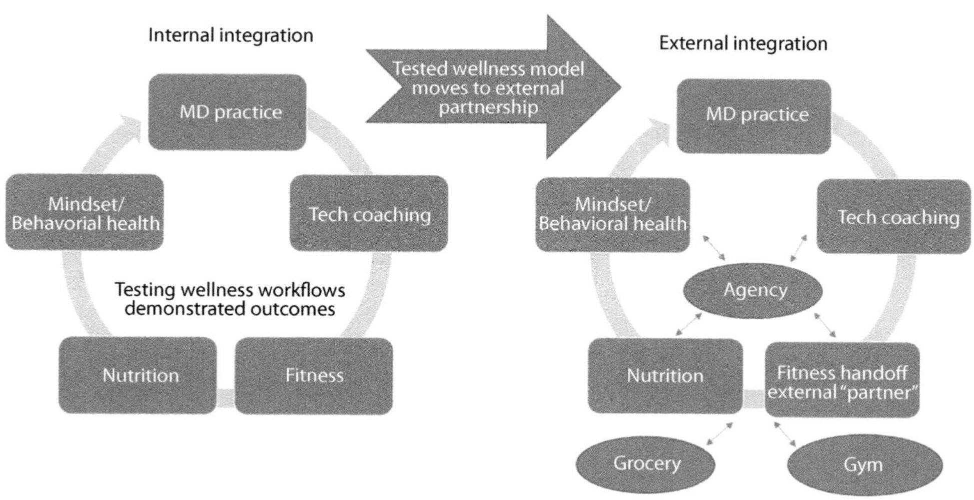

Figure 1.2 Care of health ecosystem.

Use case 1: American Heart Association: Check. Change. Control.

The American Heart Association (AHA) recently published new guidelines for hypertension management providing a spectrum of values for clinicians to manage against (Figure 1.3).[13] The agency uses these guidelines in the application of a proactive hypertension prevention and reduction process called "Check. Change. Control."[14] The program has a stand-alone application where the user can enter his or her blood pressure data over time to track performance. The AHA recently partnered with health systems and local businesses in target markets in a coordinated effort to help reduce blood pressure in target populations within an employer subpopulation. The effort has had some early success in reducing blood pressure in target populations that have successfully completed the program. The goal for the employer, long term, is to raise awareness and reduce the probability that the employee will have a cardiovascular event or die prematurely of cardiovascular disease while still employed. This presents the employer with an overt, measurable opportunity to reduce cardiovascular-related claims experience and expense over time. It presents the employee with the opportunity to lead a healthy, higher-quality, and productive life. Healthcare data is generated for analysis but is generally not integrated with other nodes of care in a healthcare system.

With the advent of wearables and smart devices, the ability to monitor blood pressure, the first step to being precontemplative regarding ones' own health, has been significantly improved. Arguably, the need of having to go to the primary

Blood Pressure Categories

American Heart Association | American Stroke Association.

BLOOD PRESSURE CATEGORY	SYSTOLIC mm Hg (upper number)		DIASTOLIC mm Hg (lower number)
NORMAL	LESS THAN 120	and	LESS THAN 80
ELEVATED	120 – 129	and	LESS THAN 80
HIGH BLOOD PRESSURE (HYPERTENSION) STAGE 1	130 – 139	or	80 – 89
HIGH BLOOD PRESSURE (HYPERTENSION) STAGE 2	140 OR HIGHER	or	90 OR HIGHER
HYPERTENSIVE CRISIS (consult your doctor immediately)	HIGHER THAN 180	and/or	HIGHER THAN 120

heart.org/bplevels

Figure 1.3 Applying class of recommendation and level of evidence to clinical strategies, interventions, treatments, or diagnostic testing in patient care* (Updated August 2015). (From Whelton, P. K. et al. *Journal of the American College of Cardiology*, 2017, doi: 10.1016/j.jacc.2017.11.006.)

care physician once per year to learn of one's own blood pressure and digest the implications given a family history in a 15-minute conversation has been altered with technology. Now, a patient can go to Amazon Prime, buy a digital blood pressure device, a heart rate device, a pulse oximeter, a scale, etc., have them delivered to the home next day, and begin using them at will, every day, multiple times a day, generating healthcare data.

Another device, the higi Station, a free-standing health screening station, is being placed in various locales, such as grocery stores, to afford users easy access where they spend a significant amount of time every week (significant being defined as one to two times per week) shopping for food. In addition to blood pressure, the higi Station captures heart rate and weight.[15] If the user creates an account, other metrics such as height and age are added, which allows users to learn their crude body mass index (BMI), another key hypertension primary prevention indicator. More healthcare data is created.

In addition to AHA and other professional medical societies, the U.S. Preventive Services Task Force (USPSTF) has created a host of recommendations on screening standards for primary prevention. The USPSTF recommends annual screening for adults aged 40 years or older and for those who are at increased risk for high blood pressure. Persons at increased risk include those who have high-normal blood pressure (130–139/85–89 mm Hg), those who are overweight or obese, and African Americans. Adults aged 18–39 years with normal blood pressure (<130/85 mm Hg) who do not have other risk factors should be rescreened every 3–5 years. The USPSTF recommends rescreening with properly measured office blood pressure and, if blood pressure is elevated, confirming the diagnosis of hypertension with ambulatory blood pressure monitoring.[16] The purpose here is not to analyze the varied recommendations from agencies, such as AHA or USPSTF, for blood pressure screening being contemplated to arrive at an evidence-based unified standard. Arguably that need does exist, and more research and consensus building in the medical community should continue in earnest. The purpose is to point out that data is being generated at multiple nodes, none of which speak to one another, but if connected could enable the healthcare analyst to determine the significance of trends and hot spots.[17]

What if we were to think about this analysis from an ecosystem point of view? The opportunity can be addressed by thinking about management of hypertension in a sub-ecosystem composed of the primary care physician, the grocery store, and wearables/devices. All three nodes can be connected with an application programming interface (API), which provides a set of clearly defined methods of communication between various software components allowing for the exchange and centralization of data, presuming the customer authorizes the exchange. The nodes can be connected by implementing the Fast Healthcare Interoperability Resources (FHIR, pronounced "fire") standard that has emerged from the nonprofit Health Level Seven International (HL7) organization, and functions as a universal adaptor allowing certain clinically relevant data types to be shared easily and securely. Most major electronic health record (EHR) vendors, such as Cerner and

Epic, have signed onto this concept and have agreed to support an early effort at implementation, known as the Argonaut Project.[18,19]

If we were able to connect the nodes, which is being done in some health systems, the healthcare analyst, in this example perhaps a health coach, will be able to review the performance data of the patient, analyze meaningful trends, curate the information, and provide it to both the patient and the primary care physician within the EMR/patient portal environment. At every annual physical, the primary care physician can review the coaching note. Ideally, when the first blood pressure reading that is taken is out of range, regardless of which standard the medical group governing evidence-based medicine at the location adopts, the primary care physician would have written an electronic order for the health coach to meet with the patient. The intervention of the health coach can be monitored over time, engagement fostered, and health outcomes improved, using data analytics.

Use case 2: Grocery store

Managing weight is a function of diet and exercise. However, the opportunity to actively manage the former at the point of contemplation has yet to be addressed at scale from a care of health perspective. What if we were to create a data node of interaction at the point of buying food that could be connected to the primary care, the wearable/device, and the fitness nodes? Building on the previous use case, the primary care physician may write an electronic order to the pre-obese patient to engage with a dietician to develop a plan. The order may require the patient to meet with his or her dietician at the grocery store, where the patient visits one to two times per week, on average. Or, the order may require the patient to meet virtually with the dietician on a telemedicine platform of choice while they plan their meal to be delivered to the doorstep the next day. Meetings with the dietician are tracked in the EMR, purchases are tracked through a loyalty database at the grocery store, and behaviors are tracked through a virtual patient journal. The dietician documents the patient's progress over time, shares the note with the health coach, who then summarizes activities for the primary care physician. Some of this work is taking place in partnerships between health systems and grocery providers. The intervention of the health coach can be monitored over time, engagement fostered, and health outcomes improved, using data analytics.

Use case 3: Exercise facility

Consider the opportunity to introduce fitness into the ecosystem. Here, the health coach expands his or her role beyond blood pressure management and diet to include a fitness regimen. Applying behavioral health and motivation principles, the health coach receives an order from the primary care physician to engage with the pre-obese patient with a family history of cardiovascular disease, diabetes, and depression. The coach meets with the patient and the dietician in the grocery store, or virtually, to develop a care plan. Progress is documented over time, and the health coach shares the summary with the primary care physician. Progress in the note is compared to height, weight, and lab values at the subsequent annual physical, and an objective conclusion is reached: either the patient made progress against goal or did not since the last annual physical. At this point, if not, a medication course may be undertaken to augment other prevention efforts. If yes, the patient goes on to live another health productive year until the next physical.

Social media and its application

Facebook is the third largest country in the population.[20] When thinking about engagement, social media cannot be ignored. Social media node(s) are ubiquitous, and depending on the age demographic, users are engaging with one another, whether texting, posting, sharing listening, favorite-ing, blogging, e-mailing, or just looking. Using the medium to leverage engagement and generate more consumer data, whether active or passive, is another opportunity for analytical use case development.

Virtual epidemiology

Investigative reporting is much like traditional epidemiological analysis of an outbreak. Just as reporters investigate an issue by investigating and verifying sources, so does the epidemiologist. In an era of social media, this aspect of investigative reporting has taken on a new dimension: individuals are reporting the early indicators of a potential outbreak before agencies who monitor disease, such as the Centers for Disease Control and Prevention, officially report the outbreak. For example, individuals experiencing symptoms of flu may search online offerings for lessening the symptoms with products such as Tamiflu or Airborne. They may search online for telemedicine offerings to consult with physicians on telemedicine platforms, such as American Well or MDOnline. This online search activity generates data and patterns for the investigative epidemiologist.

Rocky Mountain spotted fever

Consider Rocky Mountain spotted fever (RMSF), a tick-borne disease. RMSF has been a nationally notifiable condition since the 1920s. As of January 1, 2010, cases of RMSF are reported under a new category called Spotted Fever Rickettsiosis (SFR). It is well documented that the incidence of the disease is increasing over time (Figure 1.4).[21]

However, even though there is an established rise in the incidence, there may yet still be underreporting of the disease due to a multitude of factors, including patient symptom awareness, physician diagnosis awareness, insurance coverage of lab tests, etc. Reporting varies by state but arguably is reflective of the vectors influencing the spread of the disease, such as tick-carrying deer, which are more prevalent in the Midwest and mid-South (Figure 1.5).

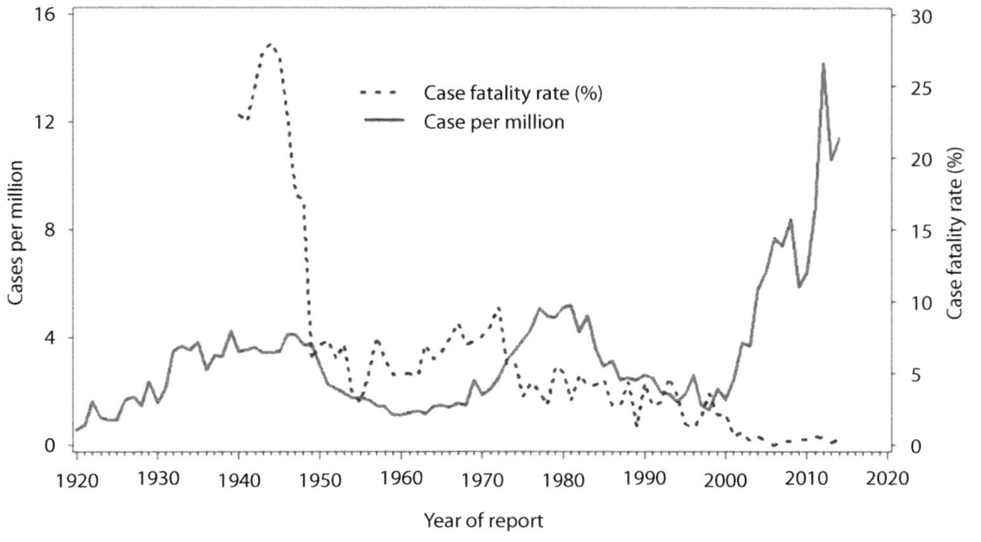

Figure 1.4 Reported incidence and case fatality of SFR in the United States, 1920–2014. Cases of SFR have been recorded since the 1920s. Trends in SFR incidence vary over time, but are generally increasing. Periods of increased incidence can be seen between 1930 and 1950 and 1968 through 1990. More recently, there has been a dramatic increase in incidence of SFR increasing from 1.7 cases per million persons in 2000 to an all-time high of 14.2 cases per million persons in 2012. Case fatality rates vary from year to year, but have had an overall decreasing trend from 28% case fatality in 1944 to less than 1% case fatality beginning in 2001.

Through an online search of nonspecific symptoms of the disease, such as high fever, chills, severe headache, muscle aches, nausea and vomiting, restlessness, and insomnia, one may aggregate symptom data with more timeliness than a public health agency relying on publically reported diagnosis through labs, public health departments, and physician offices. The challenge, of course, is that because the early symptoms of SFR are so much like other illnesses, such as the flu, one may not be able to conclusively determine that online search activity is predictive of an SFR outbreak. Online search data aggregators, such as Google analytics, can be used to monitor online chatter and plot volumes of symptom-related chatter as early indicators of an outbreak. Analysis can marry online search data with clinical diagnosis data to establish patterns and trends.

Flu

During the 2008–2009 H1N1 flu outbreak, patterns in emergency room and immediate care utilization were noticed that were race/ethnicity specific. Higher proportions of Hispanic patients were being treated from what they thought may be H1N1, a false perception largely promoted by news media indicating that those who

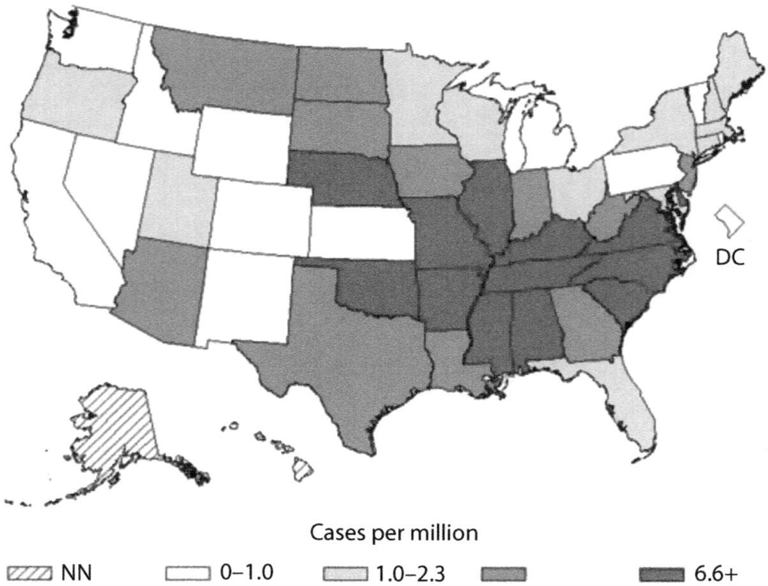

Figure 1.5 Incidence (per million population) for SFR in the United States for 2014. (NN = Not notifiable.) This figure shows the reported incidence of SFR cases by state in 2014 per million persons. SFR was not notifiable in Alaska and Hawaii in 2014. The incidence rate was reportedly zero for the District of Columbia, Kansas, Michigan, Rhode Island, Vermont, and Wyoming. Incidence ranged between 0.1 to 1.0 case per million persons for California, Colorado, Idaho, Maryland, Nevada, Ohio, Pennsylvania, and Washington. Annual incidence ranged from 1.0 to 2.3 cases per million persons in Connecticut, Florida, Maine, Massachusetts, Minnesota, New Hampshire, New York, Oregon, Utah, and Wisconsin. Annual incidence ranged from 2.3 to 6.6 cases per million persons in Arizona, Georgia, Indiana, Iowa, Louisiana, Montana, New Jersey, North Dakota, South Carolina, South Dakota, Texas, and West Virginia. The highest incidence rates, ranging from 6.6 to 278 cases per million persons were found in Alabama, Arkansas, Delaware, Illinois, Kentucky, Mississippi, Missouri, Nebraska, North Carolina, Oklahoma, Tennessee, and Virginia.

had traveled to Mexico were at higher risk. Notices of the first conformed H1N1 cases in Mexico along with signs and symptom updates were transmitted via e-mail alert by various agencies in late April 2009. By the time the World Health Organization (WHO) announced its decision to raise the Pandemic Alert Level of Phase 4 on April 27, 2009, clinical staff were already having to improvise protocols due to the pace of the spread of the outbreak locally.[22] Internal health system data aggregation, combined with geographic information system (GIS) software was used to identify utilization patterns and hot spots to allow for more targeted community education and steerage to appropriate levels of care.

At the time, telemedicine was not readily available, and many fewer social media outlets existed. Today there are apps designed to track social media chatter across multiple channels and then aggregate the information to educate the user.[23] With the most recent flu outbreak of 2017–2018 (a particularly aggressive season), the lessons of generating community awareness of the importance of vaccination and creating herd immunity, particularly among the most vulnerable, were arguably a missed opportunity. Herd immunity is a form of indirect protection from infectious disease that occurs when large proportions of population have become immune to an infection, thereby providing a measure of protection for individuals who are not immune. Combining a technology that aggregates data that is predictive of a potential outbreak with the epidemiological principal of immunization along health system utilization data could potentially prepare populations for future flu outbreaks and perhaps help to limit the spread of these outbreaks.

Reviews

With the advent of various search/purchasing platforms, such as Amazon, Yelp, Google Review, etc., consumers now review a multitude of goods, including healthcare. Reviews afford the managerial epidemiologist with a rare, real-time, data set allowing for immediate intervention. Applying principles of behavior change to social media, one can potentially harness the engagement engine of social media to improve health outcomes by pairing the two.

At one healthcare system, a proactive review process has been established to procure consumer insights in two data nodes: urgent care and the primary care physician's office (Figures 1.6 and 1.7). Prior to implementing the process, both offerings had passive engagement from a review perspective. Volumes for urgent care, for example, were averaging between 15 and 27 comments with a relatively even distribution of positive, neutral, and negative ratings. Subsequent to launching an effort asking patients for their comments post-visit, the proportion of positive reviews increased substantially as did the average rating. A by-product of the effort was the ability to monitor trends, in real-time fashion, as consumers posted comments during their encounters. For example, during the flu outbreak of 2017–2018, reviews originating from emergency rooms and urgent care centers experiencing higher than normal volumes were observed in real-time fashion, affording management with the opportunity to intervene immediately by load balancing their network of sites. In the primary care setting, systems with large medical groups spanning multiple locations can use the platform to monitor microtrends in medical offices, allowing management to intervene immediately.

A future analytical opportunity may come from the ability to leverage social media engagement with behavioral change models. Not only can we capture encounter reviews, but we can also monitor patient engagement across multiple social media platforms in target populations. One model argues that behavior change is a function of motivation, ability, and a trigger.[24] As one moves higher on the motivation curve and the change becomes easier to accomplish, a trigger can then be used to enable

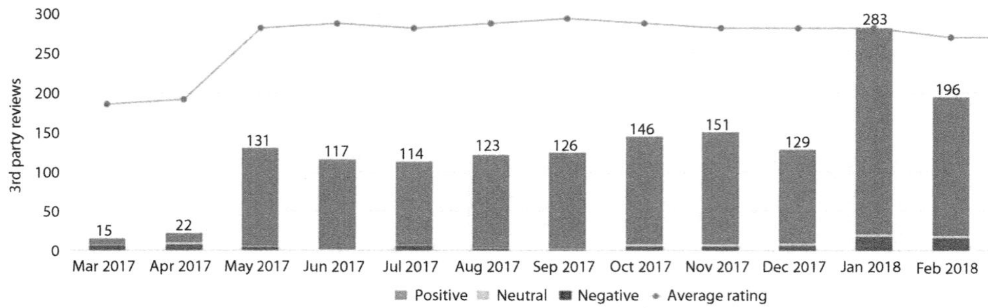

Figure 1.6 Urgent care reviews and ratings.

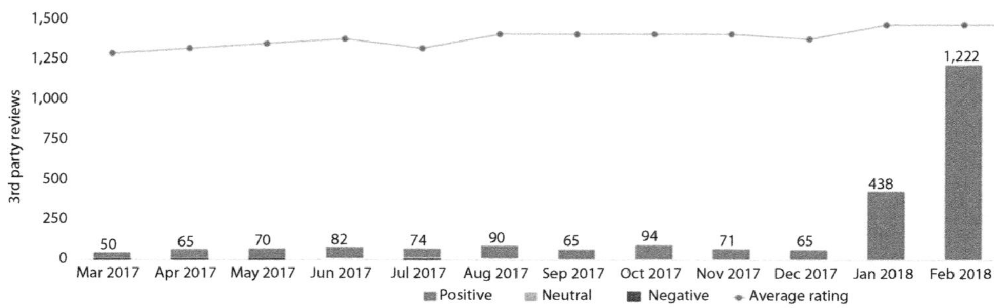

Figure 1.7 Primary care reviews and ratings.

the target behavior. There are three core motivators: sensation, anticipation, and belonging. There are two paths to increasing ability. One is that you can train people, giving them more skills, more ability to do the target behavior. The other, better path is to make the target behavior easier to do. Finally, triggers can be external or internal from a daily routine, and there are three types—facilitator, signal, and spark—according to Dr. BJ Fogg. Fogg uses Facebook as his use case example when explaining the model.

With the addition of patient engagement on social media platforms, we have the opportunity to complete the healthcare ecosystem, wrapping the healthcare provider, along with agency, grocery, and fitness with social media nodes (Figure 1.8). The data set that is created within this ecosystem affords the healthcare analyst the ability to query the data node cloud on target populations to determine the effectiveness of health improvement strategies and initiatives.

Conclusion

There is a significant amount of work yet to be done in data standardization, both in governing technology such as FHIR, and evidence-based prevention standards

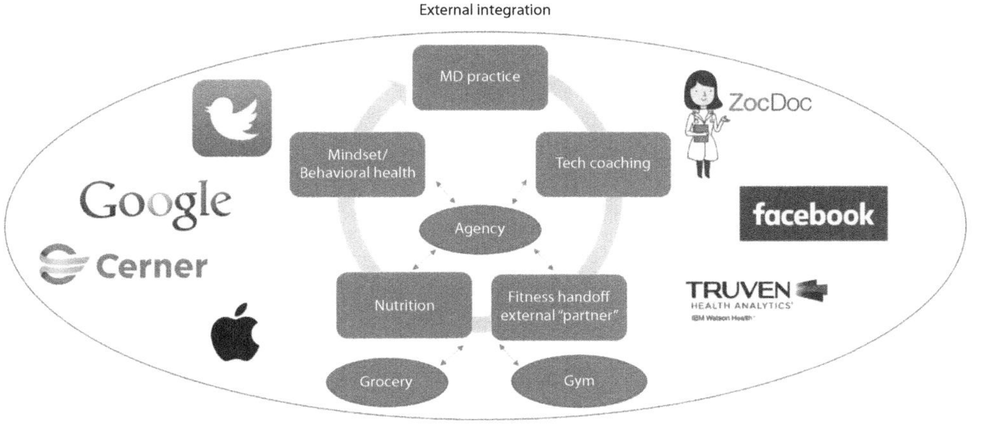

Figure 1.8 Care of health ecosystem.

such as blood pressure monitoring for hypertension. However, we are reaching an inflection point in the journey that is enabling the healthcare analyst to leverage a vast amount of data—the ability is palpable. The convergence of systems of health through partnerships that enable scaled solutions in large communities has also contributed to this inflection point. The emergence of scaled computing solutions and knowledge aggregators, such as IBM Watson Health/Truven Health Analytics and Optum/The Advisory Board Company, are also quickening the pace of analytics improvement, bringing their intellectual capital to the improvement process.

Healthcare analytics need to be flipped. Healthcare providers should ask, "What matters to you?" as well as "what's the matter?"[25,26] This flip should inform everything healthcare analysts and providers consider from a data point of view. It places the person, not the disease or the condition, at the center of improving health and healthcare within an ecosystem designed to achieve improved outcomes by meaningfully engaging with the person in a dialogue around their quality of life.[27,28] It is focused on primary prevention.

Telling the healthcare analytics story effectively requires both data art and science.[29] The ability to depict patterns in data is required from both disciplines. Software solutions, such as Tableau, allow the analyst to depict vast amounts of disparate data elegantly in one visual telling the story of health promotion and disease prevention.[30] Care of health ecosystem infographics can be built to tell a story of healthcare improvement in a community, a neighborhood, or a city. Racial and ethnic differences can be studied to better understand the underlying causes of disease.[12]

Finally, much is yet to be done to educate the healthcare analyst and equip him or her with the skills necessary to do the work. Without oversimplifying the work effort, we need to marry the technical skills of the bioinformatics professional, the investigatory skills of the epidemiologist, the mathematical skills of the statistician, the GIS skills of the cartographer, the clinical skills of the physician, the management skills of the healthcare administrator, the engagement skills of the behavioral scientist, and so on. Healthcare management curricula have not yet caught up to the need for the development of these skills, and the opportunity exists to build the academic programs of the future that will benefit society with a higher quality of life and extended life expectancy.

References

1. Fleming, S. T. 2015. *Managerial Epidemiology, Cases and Concepts*. 3rd ed. Chicago, IL: Health Administration Press.
2. Gordis, L. 2014. *Epidemiology*. 5th ed. Philadelphia, PA: Elsevier Saunders.
3. Last, J. 2000. *A Dictionary of Epidemiology*. 4th ed. New York, NY: Oxford University Press.
4. Fos, P. J., Fine, D. J. 2000. *Designing Health Care Populations: Applied Epidemiology in Health Care Administration*. San Francisco, CA: Jossey-Bass.
5. Mayzell, G. 2016. *Population Health: An Implementation Guide to Improve Outcomes and Lower Costs*. Boca Raton, FL: CRC Press.
6. George, M. L., Rowlands, D., Price, M. Maxey, J. 2005. *The Lean Six Sigma Pocket Toolbook*. New York, NY: McGraw-Hill.
7. Rafalski, E., Mullner, R. 2003. Ensuring HIPAA compliance using data warehouses for healthcare marketing. *Journal of Consumer Marketing*, 20(7), 629–633, https://doi.org/10.1108/07363760310506166
8. Rafalski, E. 2002. Using data mining/data repository methods to identify marketing opportunities in health care. *Journal of Consumer Marketing*, 19(7), 607–613, https://doi.org/10.1108/07363760210451429
9. Statistica. 2018. The Statistics Portal. Available at: https://www.statista.com/statistics/705114/amazon-services-and-products-usage-frequency-in-us/
10. Dartmouth Atlas. 2014. The Dartmouth Atlas of Health Care, Hospital Care Intensity. Available at: http://www.dartmouthatlas.org/data/table.aspx?ind=6
11. Gunderson, G., Pray, L. 2009. *Leading Causes of Life: Five Fundamentals to Change the Way You Live Your Life*. Nashville, TN: Abington Press.
12. Whitman, S. H. 2011. *Urban Health: Combating Disparities with Local Data*. New York, NY: Oxford University Press.
13. Whelton, P. K. et al. Guideline for the prevention, detection, evaluation and management of high blood pressure in adults. *Journal of the American College of Cardiology*, 2017, doi: 10.1016/j.jacc.2017.11.006
14. American Heart Association. Check. Change. Control. Community Partner Resources, 2018. Available at: http://www.heart.org/HEARTORG/Conditions/HighBloodPressure/FindHBPToolsResources/Check-Change-iControli-Community-Partner-Resources_UCM_445512_Article.jsp#.WpmJja6nFhE
15. Higi. Know your numbers. Own your health, 2018 Available at: https://higi.com
16. U.S Preventive Services Task Force. Final Recommendations Statement, 2018. Available at: https://www.uspreventiveservicestaskforce.org/Page/Document/RecommendationStatementFinal/high-blood-pressure-in-adults-screening#consider
17. Cutts, T., Rafalski, E., Grant, C., Marinescu, R. February 2014. Utilization of hot spotting to identify community needs and coordinate care for high-cost patients in Memphis, TN. *Journal of Geographic Information System (JGIS)*, 6(1), 23–29.
18. Forbes. The Last, Best Chance to Achieve Interoperability? 2016. Available at: https://www.forbes.com/sites/davidshaywitz/2016/01/18/the-last-best-chance-to-achieve-interoperability/#2e106a25643f

19. HL7 FHIR. Argonaut Project, 2017. Available at: https://www.hl7.org/documentcenter/public_temp_0F99B2F0-1C23-BA17-0CF4652D0CB8CCFA/calendarofevents/himss/2017/The%20Argonaut%20Project%20and%20HL7%20FHIR.pdf
20. The Social Media Revolution 2017. Available at: https://www.youtube.com/watch?v=PkPrZbI5C3k&t=99s
21. Centers for Disease Control and Prevention. Rocky Mountain Spotted Fever (RMSF). Available at: https://www.cdc.gov/rmsf/stats/index.html
22. Skinner, Ric. 2010. *GIS in Hospital and Healthcare Emergency Management*. Boca Raton, FL: CRC Press.
23. Sickweather. Sickness Forecasting and Mapping. Available at: http://www.sickweather.com/
24. Fogg, BJ. The Fogg Behavior Model. Available at: https://www.bjfogg.com/innovation; https://www.behaviormodel.org/
25. Bisognano, M. October 2014. Flipping healthcare: An essay by Maureen Bisognano and Dan Schumers. *BMJ*, 349, g5852, http://www.bmj.com/content/349/bmj.g5852
26. Bisognano, M. Kenney, C. 2012. *Pursuing the Triple Aim: Seven Innovators Show the Way to Better Care, Better Health, and Lower Costs*. San Francisco, CA: John Wiley and Sons.
27. Gawande, A. 2009. The Cost Conundrum. *The New Yorker*. Available at: https://www.newyorker.com/magazine/2009/06/01/the-cost-conundrum
28. Gawande, A. 2014. *Being Mortal, Medicine and What Matters in the End*. New York, NY: Metropolitan Books, Henry Holt and Company.
29. Tufte, E. R. 1991. *Visual Explanations: Images and Quantities, Evidence and Narrative*. Cheshire, UK: Graphics Press.
30. Tableau. 2018. Available at: https://www.tableau.com/

Chapter 2

Healthcare and population data: The building blocks

Razvan Marinescu with collaboration from Pradeep S. B. Podila

CONTENTS

Background

What is population health?

Kindig and Stoddart[1] define population health as "an approach [that] focuses on interrelated conditions and factors that influence the health of populations over the life course, identifies systematic variations in their patterns of occurrence, and applies the resulting knowledge to develop and implement policies and actions to improve the health and well-being of those populations"(p. 381).

They propose that population health is concerned with both the definition of measurement of health outcomes and the pattern of determinants. Determinants include medical care, public health interventions, genetics, and individual behavior, along with components of the social (e.g., income, education, employment, culture) and physical (e.g., urban design, clean air, water) environments.

The Institute for Healthcare Improvement (IHI) Triple Aim team operationally defines the term *population health* by the measures they use, noted in the "A Guide to Measuring the Triple Aim: Population Health, Experience of Care, and Per Capita Cost IHI White Paper" (2012).[2] It includes measures such as life expectancy, mortality rates, health and functional status, and disease burden (the incidence and/or prevalence of chronic disease). It also includes behavioral and physiological factors, such as smoking, physical activity, diet, blood pressure, body mass index (BMI), and cholesterol (as measured via a Health Risk Appraisal).

Recent changes in policy-level decision-making, payment structures, and provider alignment have shifted the focus from care provided and paid for at an individual level, to managing and paying for healthcare services for a discrete or defined population, an approach known as population management. The term *population management* should be clearly distinguished from *population health* (which focuses on the broader determinants of health). From the work at IHI, population management as presently practiced is best conceptualized as population medicine.[3]

Why risk stratification?

Population medicine, in this case, is the design, delivery, coordination, and payment of high-quality healthcare services to manage the Triple Aim for a population, using the best resources available within the healthcare system. The Triple Aim[4] is a framework developed by the IHI that describes an approach to optimizing health system performance. It is IHI's belief that new designs must be developed to simultaneously pursue three dimensions, which we call the "Triple Aim":

- Improving the patient experience of care (including quality and satisfaction)
- Improving the health of populations
- Reducing the per capita cost of healthcare

Much of the efforts today, such as the Accountable Care Organization (ACO), risk stratification methods, patient registries, patient-centered medical home, and other models of team-based care, are all part of a comprehensive approach to population medicine.

This chapter focuses on the risk stratification for disease states, with an example from the work performed at a large healthcare system serving patients in the U.S. mid-South region, utilizing risk stratification methodologies, to better understand complex chronic patient populations and drive their management. This region has some of the highest rates of death due to cardiovascular disease (CVD) and cancer (Figures 2.1 and 2.2) in the United States, and some of the highest prevalence rates of obesity and diagnosed diabetes (Figure 2.3) in the nation. Given this population, patients with multiple comorbidities are the norm rather than the exception. Therefore, identifying the few that drive the most expenditures is paramount to managing population health, and risk stratification is more important than ever.

Healthcare organizations working to change their cost structure and improve outcomes must design interventions that target high-risk, high-cost patients who need to be carefully and proactively managed. The success of the ACO model in delivering clinical excellence while simultaneously controlling costs depends on its ability to "incentivize hospitals, physicians, post-acute care facilities, and other providers involved to form linkages and facilitate coordination of care delivery." By increasing care coordination, ACOs can help reduce unnecessary medical care and improve health outcomes, leading to a decrease in the utilization of acute care services.

The foundational step of targeting these high-risk patients is, of course, to identify them. These patients often have multiple chronic conditions, and they are

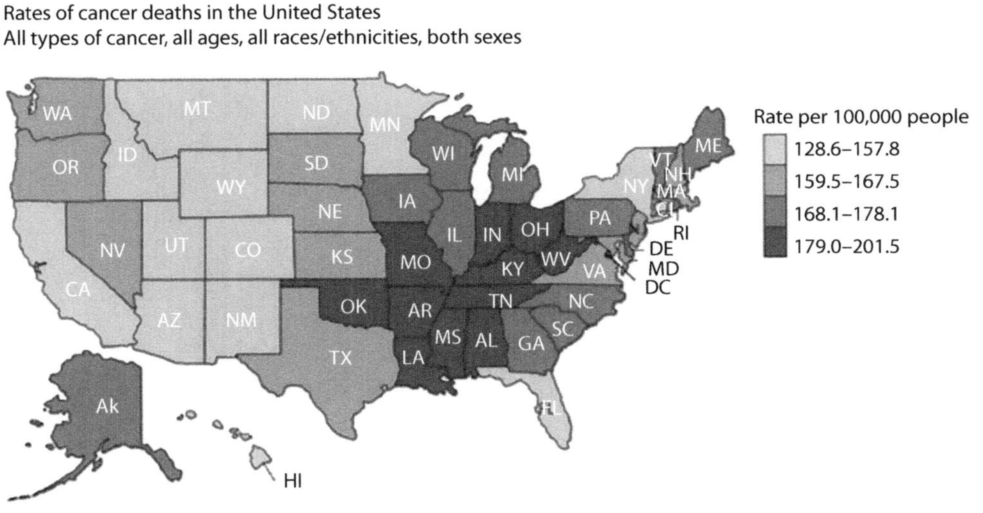

Figure 2.1 Leading cancer cases and deaths 2010–2014. (From U.S. Cancer Statistics Working Group. United States Cancer Statistics: 1999–2014 Incidence and Mortality Web-based Report. Atlanta: U.S. Department of Health and Human Services, Centers for Disease Control and Prevention and National Cancer Institute; 2017.)

likely to benefit the most from coordinating care among multiple providers and through additional community resource support. These are patients who are most at risk for significant expected health expenditures due to multiple conditions and other factors.

The process of separating patient populations into high-risk, low-risk, and the ever-important rising-risk groups is called risk stratification. It is a framework combining several individual risk scores, demographic and socioeconomic characteristics, and medical records to create a comprehensive patient profile. Furthermore, risk stratification is an integral part of care coordination, which plays a major role in ACOs and patient-centered medical home, helping hospitals manage their identified at-risk populations in such a way as to improve both patient outcomes and hospital financial performance.

With risk stratification, providers can

- Predict risks, proactively identify patients at risk of unplanned hospital admissions or readmissions.
- Develop patient-specific care plans, tailored to patient-specific risk factors.
- Understand population health trends, based on a continuous assessment and recording of risk factors.
- Support achievement of the Triple Aim: better health outcomes, quality care, and lower costs of care.

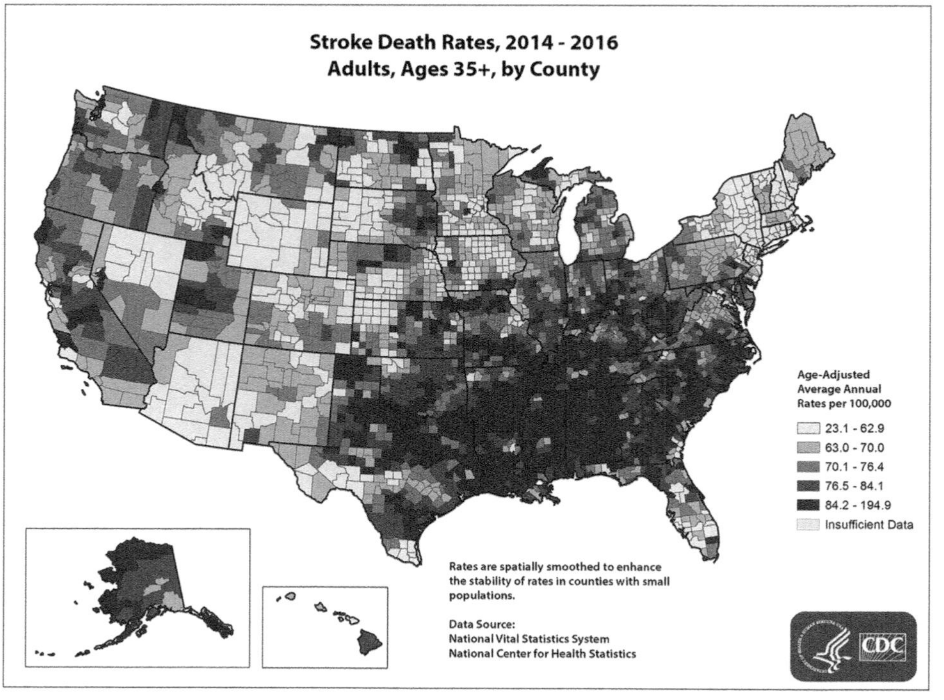

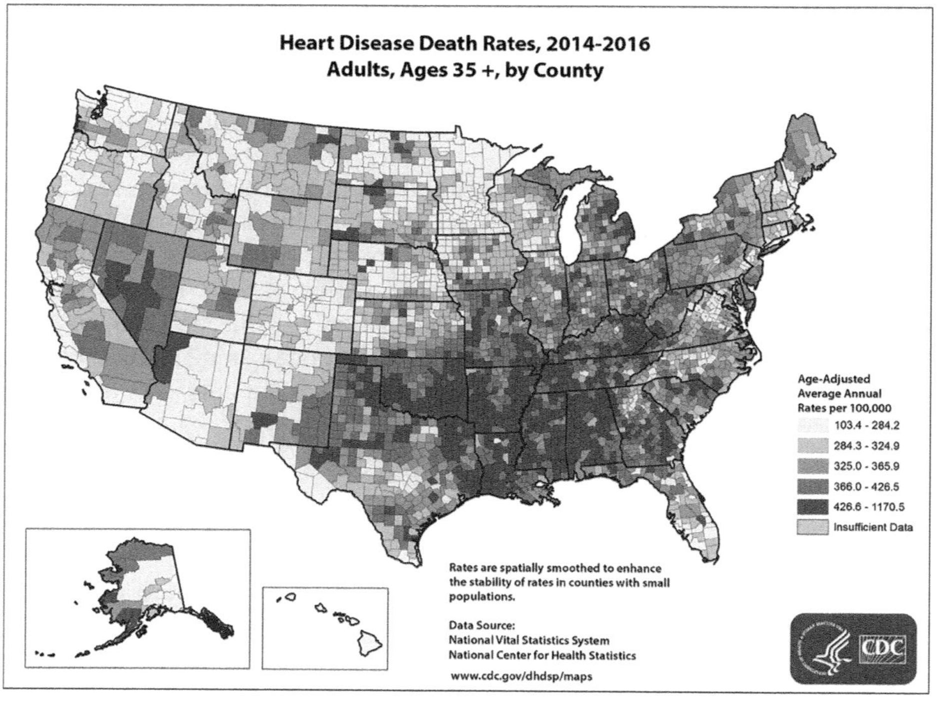

Figure 2.2 Stroke and heart disease death rates, 2013–2015, adult 65+, by county.

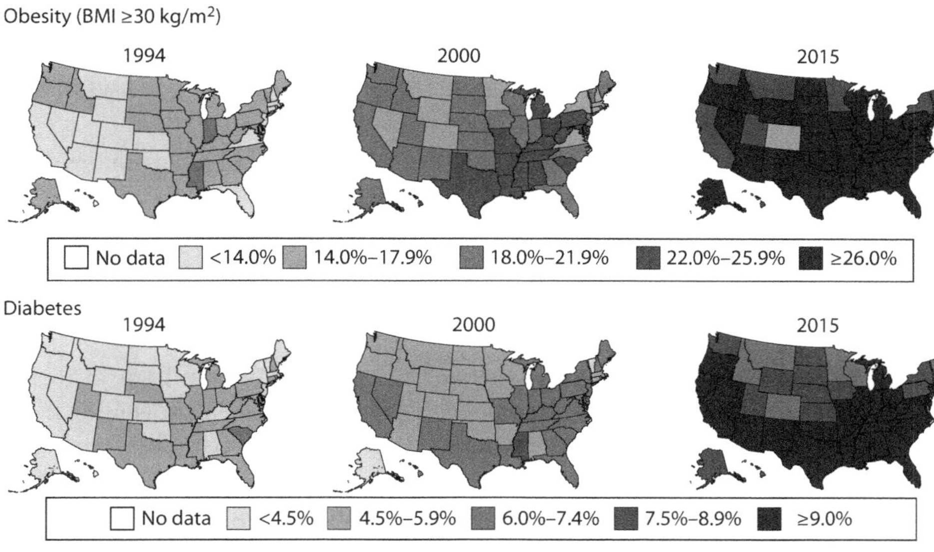

Figure 2.3 Age-adjusted prevalence of obesity and diagnosed diabetes among U.S. adults, 1994–2015. (From U.S. Department of Health and Human Services, Centers for Disease Control and Prevention; 2017.)

It is important to notice that although the terms *risk score* and *risk stratification* are sometimes used interchangeably, the two terms can have different meanings. A risk score may indicate the likelihood of a single event, such as a hospital readmission within the next 6 months, while a risk stratification framework may combine several individual risks scores, and other pertinent data, to create a broader profile of a patient.

Overview of risk stratification methods

Different organizations have proposed different health risk categories and different methodologies to bring the risk factors together. The following is an overview of several methodologies, as identified in the literature.

The American Academy of Family Physicians (AAFP)[5] proposes the following categories:

- Primary prevention (level 1 and level 2) includes patients who have low healthcare resource expenditures:
    - Patients who are healthy and have no known chronic diseases may be assigned to level 1.
    - Patients who are healthy but showing warning signs of potential health risks may be assigned to level 2.

- Secondary prevention (level 3 and level 4) includes patients who are moderate users of healthcare resources:
  - Patients who have a chronic disease but are managing it well and meeting their desired goals may be assigned to level 3.
  - Patients who are not in control of a chronic disease but have not developed complications may be assigned to level 4.

- Tertiary prevention (level 5) includes patients with high healthcare resource expenditures and whose chronic disease has progressed or become unstable, or new conditions and/or significant complications have developed.
- Catastrophic (level 6) includes patients who have extremely high healthcare resource utilization and are under the care of several subspecialties. This category is reserved for extreme situations such as a preterm baby who needs intensive long-term care, a patient with a severe head injury, or a patient requiring highly complex treatment over a relatively long period of time.

A study published in 2013 by the *American Journal of Managed Care* (AJMC) examines these six risk stratification models[6]:

- Adjusted Clinical Groups (ACGs)
- Hierarchical Condition Categories (HCCs)
- Elder Risk Assessment (ERA)
- Chronic Comorbidity Count (CCC)
- Charlson Comorbidity Index
- Minnesota Health Care Home Tiering

One thing all of these models have in common is that they are based, in some degree, on comorbidity. Understanding comorbid conditions is a critical aspect of population health management because comorbidities are known to significantly increase risk and cost. In fact, a study from the Agency for Healthcare Research and Quality reports that care for patients with comorbid chronic conditions costs up to seven times as much as care for those with only one chronic condition.[7]

In this study, while the authors are evaluating the performance of several risk-adjustment/stratification methods to predict hospitalizations, they also offer a valuable review of the main instruments to help the reader make an informed decision as to which instrument is best suited for their needs.

First, we review the study design, methods, results, and conclusions and then discuss each instrument. Next, to illustrate the process, we show the work done to identify frequent users of the Emergency Department (ED) at Methodist Healthcare, in Memphis, Tennessee (Familiar Faces [FF]), and the ensuing work to identify the rising risk population predicted to become a frequent ED user. The examples walk you through the patient cohort identification process, as well as the steps taken, and the assumptions made to identify high-risk and rising-risk patients.

Study review

The 2013 AJMC study is a retrospective cohort analysis to compare multiple methods to identify high-risk patients. Patients were 18 years and older, empaneled to the primary care clinic at Mayo Clinic, Rochester, Minnesota. Participants were assigned to a primary care provider for all 12 months in 2009 (base year) and throughout 12 months or until death in 2010 (assessment year) based on the electronic medical records that were included in the analysis. All information was electronically abstracted from the electronic medical record and administrative databases within Mayo Clinic's health records system. The study population included 83,187 patients.

Demographic variables collected in the base year included age, sex, marital status, and insurance status. Diagnosis codes (*International Classification of Diseases, Ninth Revision, Clinical Modification* [*ICD-9-CM*]) for each patient encounter, as well as utilization and cost information, were extracted from institutional billing data for year 2009. All diagnosis codes from hospitalizations, ED visits, and primary and specialty care evaluation and management visits were included.

Six models were evaluated: Adjusted Clinical Groups (ACGs), Hierarchical Condition Categories (HCCs), Elder Risk Assessment Index, Chronic Comorbidity Count, Charlson Comorbidity Index, and Minnesota Health Care Home Tiering.

Logistic regression models using demographic characteristics and diagnoses from 2009 were used to predict healthcare utilization and costs for 2010 with binary outcomes (ED visits, hospitalizations, 30-day readmissions, and high-cost users in the top 10%), using the C statistic and goodness of fit among the top decile.

Results show the ACG model outperformed the others in predicting hospitalizations. When predicting the top 10% highest-cost users, the performance of the ACG model was good and superior to the others. However, the authors conclude that although ACG models generally performed better in predicting utilization, use of any of these models will help providers implement care coordination more efficiently.

Instrument reviews and discussions

- *Adjusted Clinical Groups (ACGs)*: Developed at Johns Hopkins University to measure morbidity,[8] ACGs uses both inpatient and outpatient diagnoses to classify each patient into one of 93 ACG categories with similar expected utilization patterns. It is commonly used to predict the utilization of medical resources using the presence or absence of specific diagnoses from both inpatient and outpatient services for a specified period of time, along with age and sex. They have been found to predict inpatient hospitalizations as well as or better than other case-mix tools in many health systems.[9]
- *Hierarchical Condition Categories (HCCs)*: Part of the Medicare Advantage Program for CMS, HCCs contain 70 condition categories that contribute to a

single risk score, aggregated from *ICD-9-CM* diagnoses codes and demographic data for each patient, and include expected health expenditures.[10] Several studies among Medicare patients have provided evidence that HCCs' scores for risk adjustment can be effective at predicting hospitalizations.[11,12]

- *Elder Risk Assessment (ERA) Index*: Used to identify patients at risk for hospitalization for adults over 60 years old, the ERA index incorporates a weighted score for age, gender, marital status, number of hospital days over the prior 2 years, and selected comorbid medical illness (diabetes, coronary artery disease, congestive heart failure, stroke, chronic obstructive pulmonary disease, and dementia).[13] The minimum score on the index is –1, and the maximum score possible is 34.
- *Chronic Comorbidity Count (CCC)*: The CCC method was derived by Naessens and colleagues[14] from a modification of the method of Hwang and colleagues,[15] based on the publicly available information from the Agency for Healthcare Research and Quality (AHRQ) Clinical Classification Software. CCC is the total sum of selected comorbid conditions grouped into six categories: 0, 1, 2, 3, 4, and 5 or more. The CCC method is more comprehensive than most comorbidity counts. Comorbidity counts have been shown to be associated with high annual costs as well as persistence in high costs.[11,12]
- *Charlson Comorbidity Index*: The Charlson model sums weights for 17 specific conditions and predicts the risk of 1-year mortality for patients with a range of comorbid illnesses.[16] Based on administrative data, the model uses the presence/absence of 17 comorbidity definitions and assigns patients a score from 1 to 20, with 20 being the more complex patients with multiple comorbid conditions. It is effective for predicting future poor outcomes. The performance of the Charlson Comorbidity Index in predicting poor outcomes has been assessed in various large populations, and its validity as a prognostic measure of outcomes has been consistently demonstrated.[17]
- *Minnesota Health Care Home Tiering*: MN Tiering groups patients into "complexity tiers" based on the number of major condition categories from which they suffer.[18] Based on a product from ACGs, major expanded diagnosis clusters (MEDCs),[16] the total sum of conditions is grouped into the following five patient complexity levels: Tier 0 (Low: 0 conditions), Tier 1 (Basic: 1–3), Tier 2 (Intermediate: 4–6), Tier 3 (Extended: 7–9), and Tier 4 (Complex: 10+ conditions).

Risk stratification: Examples

Familiar Faces

Purpose

The shifts from episodic to value-based care has pushed health systems toward a proactive approach to population health needs, especially those responsible for a high percentage of total health system costs. Successful risk-based contracting and ACO development require special attention paid to patients with comorbidities and multiple visits to the ED. Building off the hot-spotting work Methodist Healthcare completed in 2012 in zip code 38109 (Memphis, Tennessee), the decision was made to pilot a program to test its ability to manage the health of a small group of high-risk individuals living in the previously identified zip code.

In 2006, Methodist Le Bonheur Healthcare (MLH) created the Congregational Health Network (CHN) that worked closely with clergy in the most underserved zip codes of the city to improve access to care and overall health status of the population.

Because the mid-South region has some of the highest prevalence rates of chronic disease, such heart disease, stroke, lung disease, cancer, diabetes, and asthma, in an effort to identify ways to improve the health of its community, MLH used geocoding technology to identify hot spots of healthcare utilization. The goal was to identify geographic areas of focus on which to direct hospital resources in a targeted effort to improve the health of the neediest communities.

The result was the identification of zip code 38109 in South Memphis. Patients from this zip code had the highest utilization of MLH EDs as well as the highest consumption of hospital charitable care. These techniques were coupled with the community health needs assessment process at MLH and qualitative, participatory research findings captured in collaboration with church and other community partners. The methodology, which we call *participatory hot-spotting*, is based on the Camden Model, which leverages hot-spotting to assess and prioritize community need in the provision of charity care but adds a participatory, qualitative layer, represented by the CHN.

Methodology

Spatial analysis was employed to evaluate hospital-based inpatient and outpatient utilization and define costs of charity care for the health system by area of residence. The top 10 zip codes accounted for 56% of total system charity care costs. The hot spot of utilization and cost was found to be South Memphis in one zip code, 38109. In 2010, in this zip code, inpatient (IP) volume accounts for 9% of visits, while representing almost 65% of total cost. Zip code 38109 has a high percentage of underserved persons and has only one Federally Qualified Health Center safety net clinic, serving roughly the 49,000 residents in the zip code. This zip code comprises 14% of the total Memphis population and is 97% African American.

As a first step in addressing the health needs of 38109, MLH launched an ongoing, innovative community health navigator pilot program—Familiar Faces—in January 2014.The pilot program provided additional, nonclinical support to the most frequent users of MLH EDs and tests the impact of navigator intervention on improving health behaviors and appropriate healthcare utilization among the FF cohort.

Results

The pilot cohort definition is "38109 Familiar Faces" (see Figures 2.4–2.7) and includes patients originating from zip code 38109 with 11 or more ED visits in a 12-month period (May 2012–April 2013). Pediatric patients were excluded. These patients had the highest utilization of EDs during the measurement period and are characterized by high rates of chronic comorbid disease.

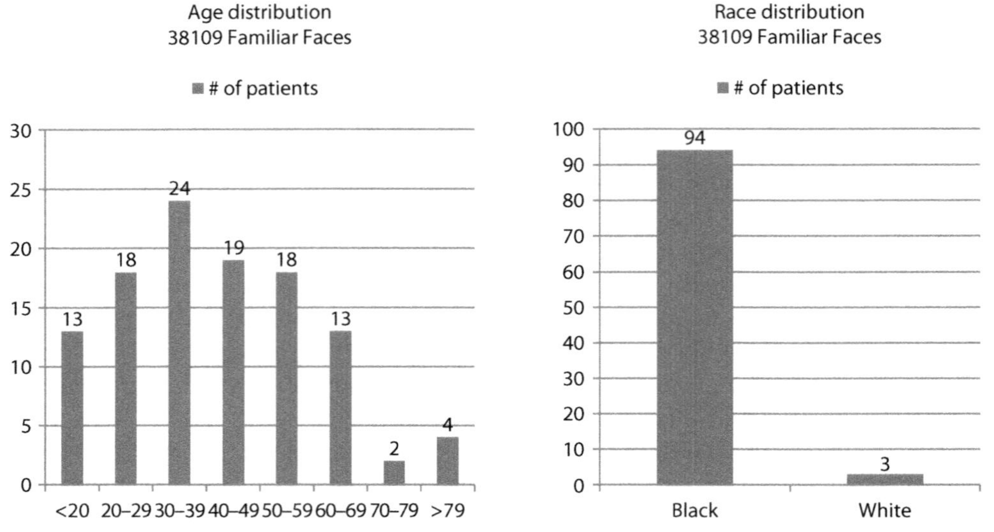

Figure 2.4 Familiar Faces age and race distribution. The largest age group in 38109 Familiar Faces is 30–39; 97% are African American. *Note:* Age distribution patient total is greater than 97 because several patients moved between groups during the specified analysis period (May '12–Sept '13). (From Ascent, Costflex May 2012–September 2013.)

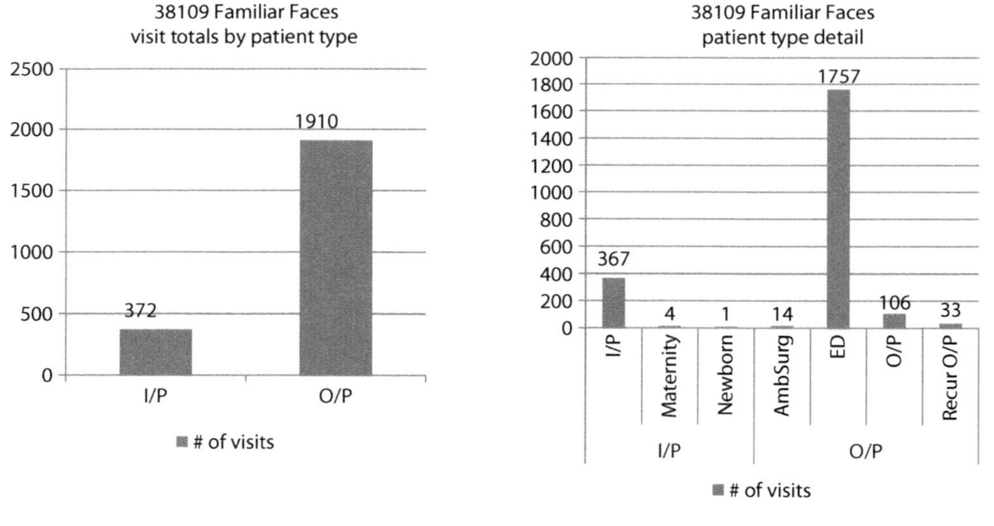

Figure 2.5 38109 Familiar Faces visits by type of patient. 38109 Familiar Faces visit our EDs on average about once per month. (From Ascent, May 2012–September 2013.)

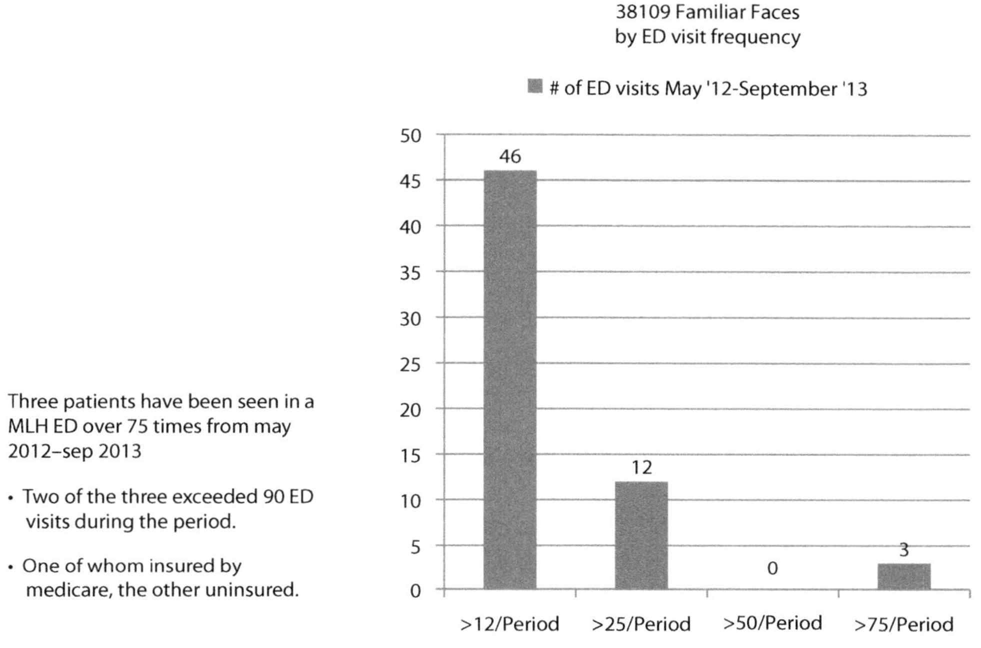

Figure 2.6 38109 Familiar Faces ED visits frequency. 46/97 Familiar Faces visited an MLH ED more than 12 times from May 2012–September 2013. (From Ascent, May 2012–September 2013.)

Total visits	Total charges	Total cost	Tot act reimb
2,282	$14,577,584	$3,439,109	$3,424,180

- 38109 Familiar Faces account for $3.4M total cost.
- Top 15 highest cost patients contribute 50% of total group cost; 8 of which are tenncare patients.
- Medicare reimbursement floats this group.
- Majority of cost comes from the IP volume.

Figure 2.7 38109 Familiar Faces costs. (From Ascent, Costflex May 2012–September 2013.)

The most common diagnoses for the FF—a group of about 100 patients—was heart failure, chronic obstructive pulmonary disease, diabetes, hypertension, and chronic kidney disease. Patients with chronic kidney disease and hypertension had the highest hospital encounter rates in this cohort. Additionally, this group had a shockingly high 2013 all-cause readmission rate approaching 60% at MLH hospitals.

Results (April 2015) showed a continuous decline in the average length of stay and the number of visits per month across the board (i.e., inpatient, ED, and outpatient encounters). In this first cohort, we have seen a 46% reduction in the cost per patient when compared to 2013 baseline and 2014 data.

Comorbidity analysis for Familiar Faces cohort

We used the following methodology to identify comorbidities in the FF cohort (see Figure 2.8): encounters for the FF cohort (2,250 total encounters) cluster around ED visits (1,618 encounters, 71.91% of total encounters) and IP visits (351 encounters, 15.6% of total), with the majority in the ED visits. Comorbidities analysis was conducted on three groups: all encounters, ED encounters, and IP encounters. Readmissions analysis was conducted on inpatient encounters after the hospice and same-day readmissions were excluded.

Results show the following (see Figure 2.9):

- Approximately 50% of the encounters had between one and five comorbid conditions associated with the principal diagnosis (shaded area).
- Two diagnosis codes associated with Chronic Kidney Disease stood out as the top two categories in the "Other" category.
- The maximum numbers of high-risk comorbidities were noticed in the case of those who were discharged with a primary diagnosis of Chronic Lung Disease (CLD), Heart Failure, Diabetes, and Chronic Kidney Disease.
- Of the encounters with a primary (principal) diagnosis code of Heart Failure (HF), 83% had at least two or more high-risk comorbidities.

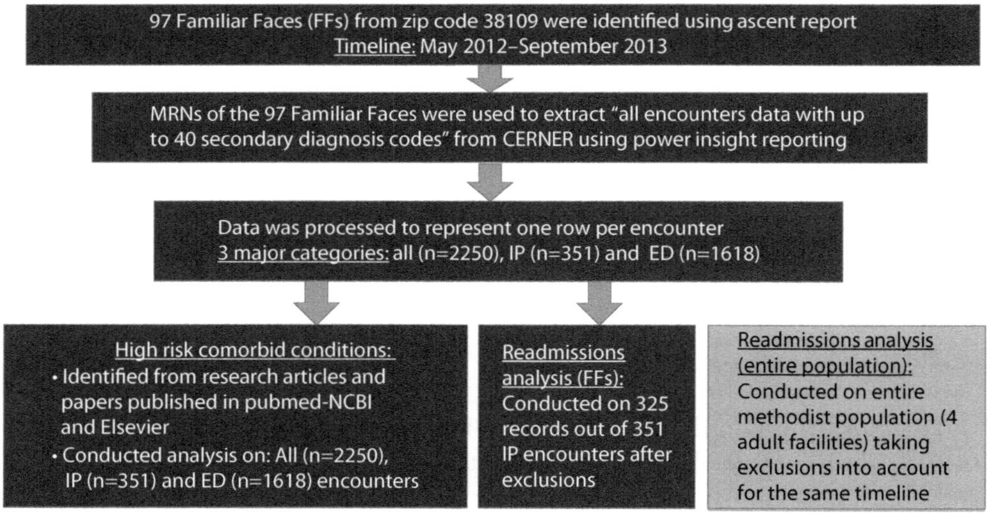

Figure 2.8 Comorbidities methodology applied to the FF cohort.

Primary diagnosis	# of comorbidities									Total
	0	1	2	3	4	5	6	7	8	
Other	891	337	258	126	70	24	8	4	2	1,720
CLD	106	28	27	18	10	4	1	1	0	195
HF	8	13	17	24	23	25	9	5	1	125
Diabetes	30	27	19	10	2	1	1	0	0	90
Sickle	44	4	2	1	1	0	0	0	0	52
PNE	6	0	2	1	1	3	3	0	0	16
ESRD	6	7	2	0	0	0	0	0	0	15
HTN	5	4	0	1	0	0	0	0	0	10
GED	6	1	0	0	0	0	0	0	0	7
AMI	1	1	0	0	0	1	1	1	0	5
CAD	1	0	0	1	2	0	0	0	0	4
Drug	1	2	1	0	0	0	0	0	0	4
Stroke	0	0	1	0	1	0	1	0	0	3
Alcohol	0	2	0	0	0	0	0	0	0	2
HIV	0	0	1	0	1	0	0	0	0	2
Total #	1,105	426	330	182	111	58	24	11	3	2,250
Total %	49.1%	18.9%	14.7%	8.1%	4.9%	2.6%	1.1%	0.5%	0.1%	

Figure 2.9 Comorbidity distribution by primary diagnosis for the FF cohort.

Readmission analysis for the Familiar Faces cohort

In terms of readmissions, the FF cohort had a significant impact on the healthcare system average readmission rate (see Figures 2.10 and 2.11):

- The FF population has a higher readmit rate than the system population.
- The highest readmission rate burden is for HF patients.

Readmission cause	FFs	EP	EP-FFs	Impact
AMI	66.67%	11.84%	11.76%	0.08%
HF	57.53%	20.99%	20.16%	0.83%
Pneumonia	37.50%	15.21%	15.14%	0.07%
All cause	52.38%	12.90%	12.72%	0.18%

Figure 2.10 All payer readmissions. (MHMH, methodist healthcare memphis hospitals [four adult facilities]; EP, entire methodist population [four adult facilities—MUH, MSH, MNH, and MGH]; FFs, 97 Familiar Faces identified from zip code 38109; EP–FFs, entire methodist population minus encounters of the 97 Familiar Faces identified from zip code 38109; Burden-EP, EP-FFs; Date range, May 2012–September 2013.)

Readmission cause	FFs	EP	EP-FFs	Impact
AMI	100.00%	14.78%	14.69%	0.09%
HF	19.91%	21.60%	20.89%	0.71%
Pneumonia	33.33%	15.47%	15.43%	0.04%
All cause	58.06%	15.90%	15.68%	0.22%

Figure 2.11 Medicare readmissions. (MHMH, methodist healthcare memphis hospitals [four adult facilities]; EP, entire Methodist population [four adult facilities—MUH, MSH, MNH, and MGH]; FFs, 97 Familiar Faces identified from zip code 38109; EP–FFs, entire methodist population minus encounters of the 97 Familiar Faces identified from zip code 38109; Burden-EP, EP-FFs; Date range, May 2012–September 2013.)

- The 30-day readmission rate was reduced by 3.15% at Methodist South Hospital (MSH) when the encounters of the 97 FFs were excluded from the entire Methodist Healthcare Memphis Hospitals (MHMH) population.
- This clearly shows the disproportionate effect of FF readmission rates on the healthcare system average.

Contribution factor Familiar Faces cohort: Rising risk identification

In order to identify rising-risk patients within the FF cohort (96 patients remaining out of the 100 in the initial cohort, due to the death of four patients), one of the methods we used was to determine a contribution factor calculated as a ratio of the number of encounters to the number of unique patients.

As seen in Figure 2.12, when we calculate the contribution factor for principal discharge diagnosis within the FF cohort (94 patients, 1,563 encounters), patients with diagnoses of Chronic Kidney Disease and Hypertension have the highest utilization rates as well as the highest factor. The contribution factor helped us identify the focus

Readmission cause	Encounters – IP & OP (Unique patients)	Contribution factor
Chronic kidney disease	35 (4)	8.75
Hypertension	83 (10)	8.3
Diabetes	59 (11)	5.36
HF	74 (18)	4.11
COPD	47 (16)	2.94
AMI	3 (3)	1
PNE	8 (8)	1
STK	2 (2)	1
Other	1,252 (94)	13.31
Total	1,563 (94)	16.63

Figure 2.12 Contribution factor in the FF cohort.

of our intervention within the cohort. Initial results show these two comorbidities are the most likely disease states to result in frequent ED and IP visits.

Rising risk methodology: Follow-up on 38109 familiar faces

Purpose

Results suggest the community navigator pilot program is working (https://pdfs.semanticscholar.org/8476/adea8f44c24bed9053cc08bc6bcc3aae3145.pdf). However, we now want to expand the program to a larger population of patients in 38109—those that are at risk of becoming a FF.[19] The next step was to extend and strengthen our support for these high-/rising-risk patients by identifying patients with the potential of becoming a FF through the expansion of navigation support to include patients who are referred to home health services for ongoing care after hospital stays, and working more closely with patients who are registered members of the Congregational Health Network.

In this example of risk stratification, we aim to

- Identify the patients who are at risk of moving into the "frequent flyers category" and of becoming FF patients (as defined by the initial cohort).
- Better assess the prevalent chronic disease conditions so that targeted population health strategies can be designed to address the issues.
- Identify comparable populations from other zip codes.
- Better prepare us for the next submission of Community Health Needs Assessment (CHNA) to maintain our not-for-profit status.

Our metrics of success are as follows:

- Reduce ED visits, hospital admissions, and cost.
- Increase the days between visits to an acute care provider.
- Manage chronic disease through successful use of telehealth products and personal support by a navigator by employing a case/control cohort prospective study design.

Methodology

The rising-risk cohort (R^2) methodology is as follows:

- To identify the R^2 cohort, we begin by analyzing the ED encounters over an 18-month period.
- We then isolate adult-only patients who originate from 38109, our hot spot zip code.

- Using Pareto analysis, we then segregate those patients who are considered a high utilization cohort, those with six or more ED encounters over an 18-month period.
- We remove those patients who expired during the study period and further refine the cohort to isolate FFs from those who are R^2, $\geq$6 and $\leq$10 ED encounters.
- Once the R^2 cohort has been identified, we stratify the group by encounter classification: ED, IP, and observation (OBS).
- We remove patients diagnosed with HIV for patient confidentiality and proceed to score the three groups based on their comorbidities, utilization patterns, and acuity/readmission/length of stay.

The patient cohort identification process is as follows:

- Identification of the final cohort for rising-risk analysis (Figures 2.13–2.16)
- Comorbidity identification and scoring
- Risk scores calculation and patient selection

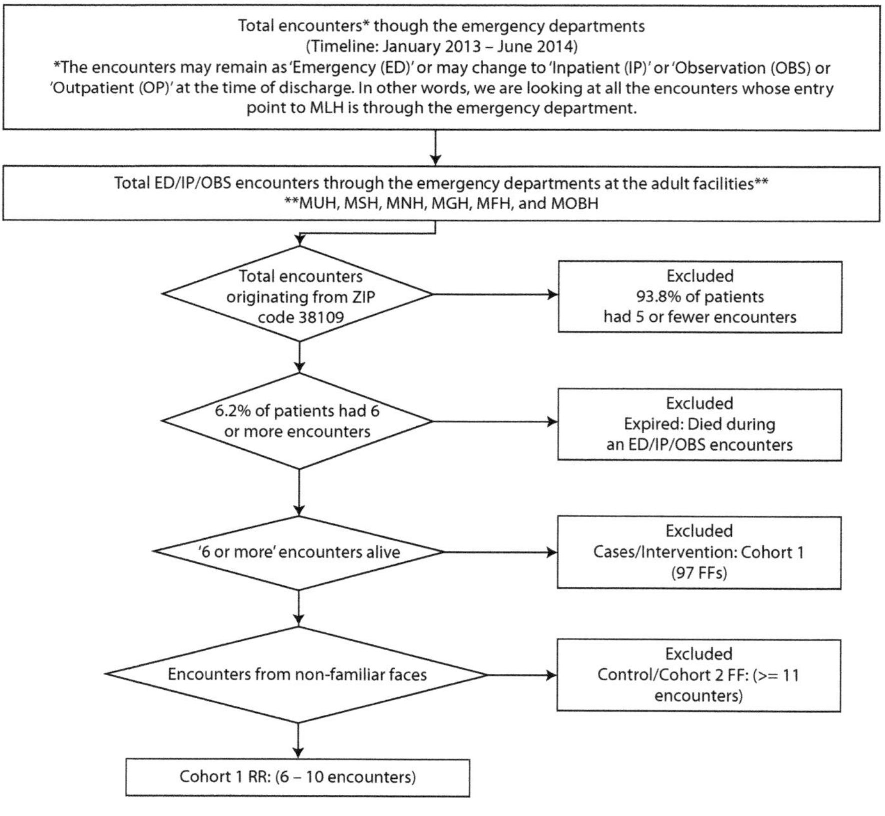

Figure 2.13 Cohort selection.

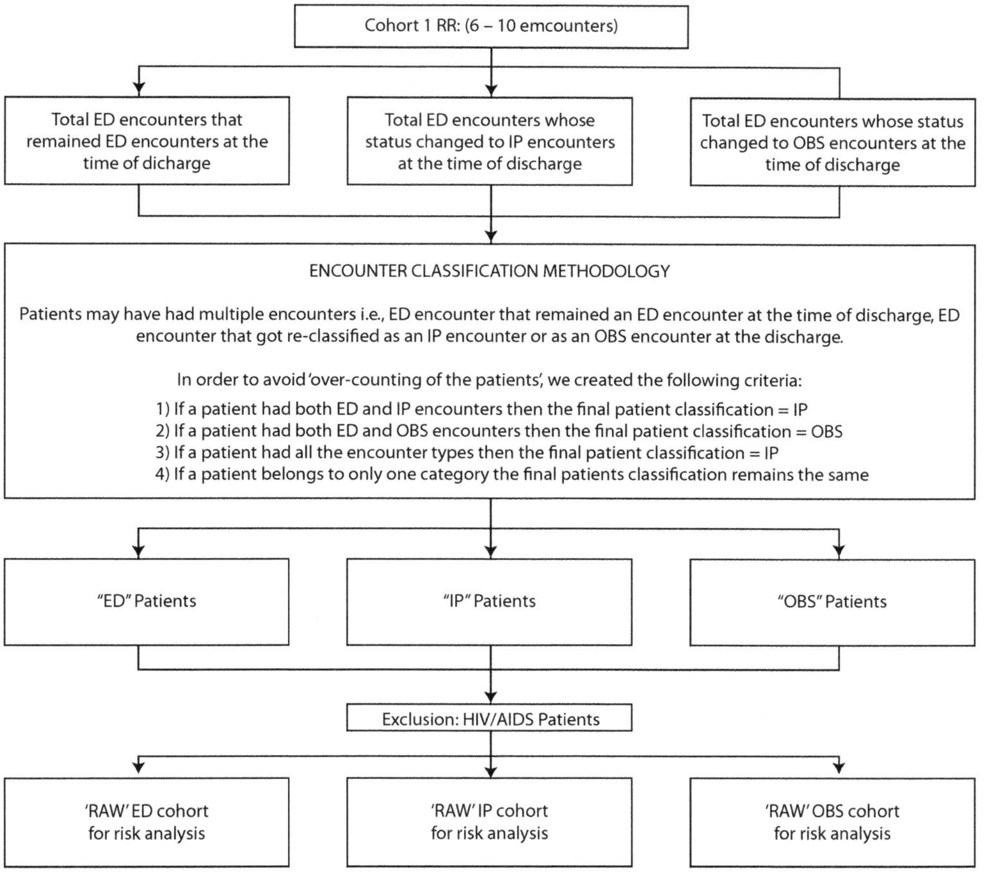

Figure 2.14 Cohort encounter classification.

Use of data

Data analytics is the current buzzword in healthcare, and rightly so. Access to actionable data combined with the right analysis helps not only in predicting outcomes, but also in improving the ability of care teams to align available resources to what a patient needs. Although data is just a start and not an endpoint, data can be used in several ways to make the process of risk stratification less cumbersome:

- *Optimal use of data*: Going beyond clinical and claims data to socioeconomic data and other relevant information that describe a patient and integrating multiple sources of information to let providers understand what works best for a patient.
- *Performing analytics*: Identification of underlying risk factors will alert providers well in time of any complication that might occur.

'Raw' ED cohort for risk analysis

'Raw' IP cohort for risk analysis

'Raw' OBS cohort for risk analysis

Run the *"comorbidity identification methodology"* on the above "Raw IP/ED/OBS Cohorts" separately using the list of disease conditions. Note: For this we have only considered the first 5 DXs in a patient's medical record.

Create a *summary record for each patient* with all the comorbidities identified in each of their encounters during the timeframe used to identify the rising risk population i.e., as long as a condition is present in one of the encounters the information will be carried forward to the summary level record. Scientifically, this seems like a better way to understand all the disease conditions a patient experienced during the timeframe selected.

Add Acuity Level (ED data), Count and Type of readmissions (IP data), and LOS (OBS data) to the summary level records. Now, apply the following scoring methodology.

Scoring Methodology: 3 Key Domains: FINAL SCORE = "Weighted Sum" of individual domain scores

Domain	ED	IP	OBS
1	ED comorbidities ➢ None = 0 ➢ 1 to 3 = 1 ➢ >=4 then 2	IP comorbidities ➢ None = 0 ➢ 1 to 3 = 1 ➢ >=4 then 2	OBS comorbidities ➢ None = 0 ➢ 1 to 3 = 1 ➢ >=4 then 2
2	ED utilization ➢ None = 0 ➢ 1 ED encounter =1 ➢ 2 to 4 ED encounter = 2 ➢ >4 ED encounter = 3	IP utilization ➢ None = 0 ➢ 1 IP admission = 1 ➢ 2 to 4 IP admissions = 2 ➢ >4 IP admissions = 3	OBS utilization ➢ None = 0 ➢ 1 OBS admission = 1 ➢ 2 to 4 OBS admissions = 2 ➢ >4 OBS admissions = 3
3	Highest ED acuity level ➢ Level 5 = 1 ➢ Level 4 = 2 ➢ Level 3 = 3 ➢ Level 2 = 4 ➢ Level 1 = 5	30-day IP readmissions ➢ None or No readmissions = 0 ➢ Any one type of IP readmission for AMI or HF OR PNE = 1 ➢ Any one type of IP readmission for AMI or HF OR PNE = 2 ➢ Any one type of IP readmission for AMI or HF OR PNE = 3	LOS-midnight rule ➢ 1 midnight (<48 hrs) = 0 ➢ 2 midnight (>=48 hrs) = 1

Figure 2.15 Comorbidity identification and scoring.

- *Monitoring growth and outcomes*: Data from previous successes and failures can help care teams redesign care plans and ensure complete patient-centric care.
- *Incorporating data into risk scores*: Creating risk scores as a blend of behavioral, demographic, and clinical data will provide physicians with a holistic view of patients to improve outcomes across the care continuum.[20]

Risk score for ED data = 1/3 (ED comorbidities) + 1/3 (ED utilization) + 1/3 (Highest ED acuity level)
Risk score for IP data = 1/3 (IP comorbidities) + 1/3 (IP utilization) + 1/3 (30-day IP readmissions)
Risk score for OBS data = 1/3 (OBS comorbidities) + 1/3 (OBS utilization) + 1/3 (LOS – midnight rule)

ED_Risk_score	/Unique patients	Frequency
1.65	15	3.36%
1.98	110	24.66%
2.31	159	35.65%
2.64	140	31.39%
2.97	22	4.93%
Grand total	446	100.00%

IP_Risk_Score	/Unique patients	Frequency
0.33	14	467%
0.66	86	28.67%
0.99	46	15.33%
1.32	98	32.67%
1.65	45	15.00%
1.98	11	3.67%
Grand total	300	100.00%

OBS_Risk_Score	/Unique patients	Frequency
0.33	19	17.76%
0.66	44	41.12%
0.99	28	26.17%
1.32	10	9.35%
1.65	6	5.61%
Grand total	107	100.00%

Select a cut-off score for each of the 3 focus areas i.e., 1) ED, 2) IP, and 3) OBS to identify the Rising Risk population

Figure 2.16 Risk scores calculation and patient selection.

References

1. Kindig, D., Stoddart, G. 2003. What is population health. *American Journal of Public Health*, 93(3).
2. Stiefel, M., Nolan, K. 2012. *A Guide to Measuring the Triple Aim: Population Health, Experience of Care, and Per Capita Cost.* IHI Innovation Series white paper. Cambridge, MA: Institute for Healthcare Improvement. Available at: http://www.IHI.org
3. Lewis, N. 2014. *Populations, Population Health, and the Evolution of Population Management: Making Sense of the Terminology in US Health Care Today.* Cambridge, MA: Institute for Healthcare Improvement. Available at: http://www.ihi.org/communities/blogs/_layouts/15/ihi/community/blog/itemview.aspx?List=81ca4a47-4ccd-4e9e-89d9-14d88ec59e8d&ID=50
4. *IHI Triple Aim Initiative.* Available at: http://www.ihi.org/Engage/Initiatives/TripleAim/Pages/default.aspx
5. Risk-stratified Care Management, available at: https://www.aafp.org/practice-management/transformation/pcmh/key-functions/care-management.html
6. Haas, L. R. et al. Risk-stratification methods for identifying patients for care coordination. *American Journal of Managed Care*, Sept. 17, 2013.
7. Just, E. 2016. *Understanding Risk Stratification, Comorbidities, and the Future of Healthcare.* Health Catalyst.
8. Weiner, J. P., Starfield, B. H., Steinwachs, D. M., Mumford, L. M. 1991. Development and application of a population-oriented measure of ambulatory care case-mix. *Medical Care*, 29(5):452–472.
9. Bernstein, R. H. 2007. New arrows in the quiver for targeting care management: High-risk versus high-opportunity case identification. *Journal of Ambulatory Care Management*, 30(1):39–51.
10. Pope, G. C. et al. 2004. Risk adjustment of Medicare capitation payments using the CMS-HCC model. *Health Care Financing Review*, 25(4):119–141.
11. Li, P., Kim, M. M., Doshi, J. A. 2010. Comparison of the performance of the CMS Hierarchical Condition Category (CMS-HCC) risk adjuster with the Charlson and Elixhauser comorbidity measures in predicting mortality. *BMC Health Services Research*, 10:245.
12. Lin, P. J., Maciejewski, M. L., Paul, J. E., Biddle, A. K. 2010. Risk adjustment for Medicare beneficiaries with Alzheimer's disease and related dementias. *American Journal of Managed Care*, 16(3):191–198.
13. Crane, S. J., Tung, E. E., Hanson, G. J., Cha, S., Chaudhry, R., Takahashi, P. Y. 2010. Use of an electronic administrative database to identify older community dwelling adults at high-risk for hospitalization or emergency department visits: The elders risk assessment index. *BMC Health Services Research*, 10:338.
14. Naessens, J. M. et al. 2011. Effect of multiple chronic conditions among working-age adults. *American Journal of Managed Care*, 17(2):118–122.
15. Hwang, W., Weller, W., Ireys, H., Anderson, G. 2001. Out-of-pocket medical spending for care of chronic conditions. *Health Aff (Millwood)*, 20(6):267–278.
16. Charlson, M. E., Pompei, P., Ales, K. L., MacKenzie, C. R. 1987. A new method of classifying prognostic comorbidity in longitudinal studies: Development and validation. *Journal of Chronic Diseases*, 40(5):373–383.
17. Li, B., Evans, D., Faris, P., Dean, S., Quan, H. 2008. Risk adjustment performance of Charlson and Elixhauser comorbidities in ICD-9 and ICD-10 administrative databases. *BMC Health Services Research*, 8:12.

18. Minnesota Department of Human Services. Health Care Homes: Minnesota Health Care Programs (MHCP) Fee-for-Service Care Coordination Rate Methodology. Available at: https://www.dhs.state.mn.us/main/idcplg?IdcService=GET_DYNAMIC_CONVERSION&RevisionSelectionMethod=LatestReleased&dDocName=DHS16_151066. Accessed July 6, 2019.
19. Podila, P. S. B. 2015. *Methodology is Copyrighted and Patent is Pending*. Memphis, TN: Methodist Le Bonheur Healthcare.
20. Shashank, A. 2017. *The Importance of Risk Stratification in Population Health Management*. HIT Consultant Media. Available at: http://hitconsultant.net/2017/03/13/risk-stratification-population-health-management/

Chapter 3

Trend toward connected data architectures in healthcare

Greg Jordan

CONTENTS

Healthcare technology professionals and administrators who are responsible for their respective organizations' data systems encounter challenges often found in other industries. Regardless of industry, any organization or company whose success is even partially dependent on data has to ensure that the systems are highly available, accurate, and precise. These needs are at the core when choosing a database, designing the data architecture, and implementing any application that will ultimately make use of the organization's data.

However, healthcare data has unique challenges when compared to other industries. Over the lifetime of a single patient, an enormous volume of data will be generated from electronic medical record (EMR) systems, imaging systems, monitoring systems, as well as the related insurance and financial systems. For example, a 2014 report from the International Data Corporation predicts that healthcare data volume will grow from 153 exabytes to more than 2,300 exabytes by 2020.[1] In just a few years, healthcare systems will create about 350 gigabytes of data for every person on the planet—equivalent to the disk capacity for the average laptop computer.

Data volume is just one of the particular challenges facing healthcare organizations. The growing amount of data is also variable and complex, the data might be well defined or unstructured, and the sources can use different data formats. To address these issues, healthcare professionals should consider three discrete areas in order to have the greatest impact within respective organizations, specifically, balancing cost and performance, mitigating risk, and connecting disparate data sources.

Balancing cost and performance

The first challenge in managing healthcare systems is increasing the value and performance while controlling the costs. At the core of the dual challenge of controlling costs and increasing value is the database. A database that can reliably, consistently, and efficiently store and retrieve hundreds of millions of records as well as support hundreds of thousands of requests from dependent applications every day comes with a high price.

First, databases often require computer hardware that is specially designed for data storage and retrieval, which means the capital cost will be higher than commodity hardware used in related and supporting systems. In order to setup, configure, and maintain a database that will perform reliably, consistently, and efficiently, organizations must hire professionals with the necessary expertise and experience. To integrate the database with standard applications, such as an EMR, additional experts will need to be hired. Further, organizations often need to create customized applications to support specific, discrete operations, which requires even more expert technology people to be hired. Finally, the database software requires purchasing support as well as a license or multiple licenses from a vendor. The cost of support and database licenses is variable but is usually determined based on how the database will be used. The initial price of obtaining the hardware, software, and people involved can result in the amount of tens of millions of dollars on an annual basis. Organizations must also support the costs that will ensure the continuity of the operations as well as make sure the system can effectively handle the eventual growth of the volume of data.

Risk management

As technology professionals working in healthcare can attest, one of the most challenging aspects of projects involving data is mitigating risk. Mitigating risk deals with carefully addressing the areas of security, structure, and design of the data. A critical part of the challenge when managing data structure and design, which can be referred to collectively as the *schema*, is reducing or eliminating risk while making additions or modifications. This risk is not necessarily unique to healthcare data systems, but the risk involved with these changes, even for what could be considered minor changes, can have a severe impact on patient outcomes as well as the cost of healthcare.

There is a subset of healthcare data-driven applications, such as accounting systems, that will have modest schema modifications over time. The inputs and outputs for those types of applications change infrequently because these were some of the earliest applications developed in healthcare settings, and it has been long understood which data is critical to the success of these applications. Therefore, changing the schema usually occurs only a few times over the lifetime of these systems.

At the other end of the spectrum, systems that can produce breakthroughs and better healthcare outcomes need frequent schema modifications. For example, when closely examining data patterns inside EMRs for a specific procedure, an analyst might eventually understand why readmission occurs less frequently in one hospital when compared to another hospital. Since these types of systems can collect the richest and most valuable data and are candidates for new analysis or modifications to existing analysis, it becomes routine for new and varied data to be added or changed. In either case of modest or frequent schema modifications, mitigating risk that can be introduced often is the highest hurdle in the race to improve the results.

Further, the type of risk is not isolated to a single area. On the contrary, the risks in schema change can take the form of one or more of the following:

- Privacy and security degradation
- Data loss
- Data corruption
- Data quality
- Increased data response times
- Application errors
- Productivity loss

Because these areas of risk can be introduced in parallel, it can compound the potential problem. Consider the following scenario: a team implements a schema change to provide a new report that shows costs for readmission rates for specialty procedures. While the change was successfully tested and added into the production reporting system, other financial reports suddenly began to display much more slowly and, in some cases, produce inconsistent information. While the project team considered rolling back the change, they instead opted to fix it. The fix required the full attention of the team and was implemented after a few days, but a few days later new errors in unrelated reports began surfacing. Finally, after several weeks, all of the application and reporting errors were resolved.

Even using best practices in security, testing, and change management, scenarios similar to the one above do happen. A number of human factors can contribute or cause these scenarios, but the constraints in the database systems can also contribute. The simple example offered here might be considered a best-case outcome that had minor failures, especially since no security issues were created, no data was lost, and, most importantly, no patients were harmed.

Teams that do not prioritize testing or follow a rigorous process for change management can, and often do, introduce issues that will not be discovered until after data breach, data corruption, or data loss has occurred. In some cases, the failure is not revealed until well after the change was made. For example, in 2003 at St. Mary's Mercy Hospital in Grand Rapids, Michigan, 8,500 patients were declared dead after a mapping error occurred during a system update.[2] The patients and the hospital were not aware of the issue until bills were sent out by the hospital's system.

Sharing and connecting data

The time, effort, and cost of setting up and maintaining data and then managing the accompanying risks are just two parts of the foundation in successful data management. The remaining challenge is ensuring that data can be shared and connected across the organization, with collaborating organizations, and with patients and caregivers. The value of data that is created and remains in one department is comparatively low as compared to data that can be shared.

When medical professionals participate in rounds or other continuing medical education, they learn new and improved ways to take better care of their patients. They connect and take part in information sharing, whether at the bedside or in the classroom, that has proven to result in measurably better outcomes. The sharing of data between computer systems should be viewed the same way. Just as valuable medical education and training follow a rigorous process and adhere to strict standards, healthcare administrators should treat the organization's valuable data similarly.

However, healthcare data often becomes siloed, which happens for a number of reasons. In one case, the data might have compliance and regulatory factors that create barriers to sharing. Data also becomes trapped in organizations that have not fostered a culture that promotes the open sharing of data. While human factors play a role in creating this culture, the specific and seemingly carefully selected data systems themselves prevent connecting and sharing data. This reason often stems from the aforementioned cost, performance, and risk inherent within data systems. For example, budget priorities might force department administrators to delay implementation of new systems or processes to share data. In addition, administrators might give greater weight to the risk involved as compared to perceived benefits.

These issues can be overcome, especially in light of newer data systems that reduce costs, increase performance, better mitigate risk, and share information. In the next sections, we review the relatively new database options that allow healthcare technology professionals and administrators to more easily achieve management and analysis advancements through shared, highly connected data. Before reviewing new options, it is important to understand the data systems that are currently in use and how they have contributed to the status quo.

Current state of databases in healthcare systems

Relational databases were first developed in the 1970s, and their origin is often credited to Edgar F. Codd, who at the time was an engineer for IBM.[3] Their widespread adoption is primarily a result of the maturity of the ecosystem of relational databases. Over the past 45 years, database vendors have created dozens of competing systems that adhere to the rules first laid out by Codd. Further, vendors have created data analysis and management tools to support those systems. The relational database has become a staple in the coursework for computer science students. With healthcare systems also beginning to come of age in the 1970s, it should then come as no surprise that healthcare applications have almost exclusively made use of a relational database as the primary data system.[4]

As shown in Figure 3.1, this data structure allows specifically named *tables* of data with rows and columns to be related to one another through keys. *Primary keys* represent the unique identifier of the row within its respective table. *Foreign keys* use the unique ID from the corresponding table or tables to create the relationships between the records. Since patients can have multiple visits, a patient visit record contains a foreign key to a single patient record.

Challenges with relational systems

While relational systems are well understood and many organizations have made significant investments toward supporting them, they struggle to truly represent the messy, complex, and real world in which patients are treated. As noted earlier, relational systems were first designed in the 1970s, and the computers from that era had vastly different limitations in processing capability, storage capacity, and performance. For example, a gigabyte of disk space—roughly enough to store 2 hours of video—in 1980 would have cost nearly $200,000, but today could be

Primary Key

Patient		
PatientID	**Fname**	**Lname**
1479743393	Clara	Jordan
1795969139	Richard	Jordan
2725848812	Andrew	Wray
3229863141	Opal	Jordan
3426178398	Nancy	Chiozza
5470739690	Alvin	Jordan
6223848281	Linda	Jordan
7154042678	Louis	Chiozza
7753708318	Aline	Wray
9557437033	Donald	Jordan

Foreign Key

Patient Visit			
VisitID	**PatientID**	**Date**	**Doctor**
1	9557437033	2005-04-21	Elizabeth
2	9557437033	2005-11-15	Kathryn
3	1479743393	2006-03-16	Donald
4	3426178398	2007-02-22	Lee Anne
5	9557437033	2007-08-13	Andrew M
6	1479743393	2008-02-27	Lou
7	2725848812	2009-01-23	Mark
8	7753708318	2009-08-13	Brian
9	7753708318	2010-05-20	Steve
10	9557437033	2011-09-13	Bill
11	3229863141	2011-11-28	Rachel
12	7154042678	2012-06-01	Gregory
13	5470739690	2013-03-04	Samuel
14	1795969139	2013-12-19	Andrew W

Figure 3.1 Example representation of a primary and foreign key relationship in a relational database.

had for $0.03.[5] These compute limitations curtailed novel ideas and forced core architecture decisions with which technology professionals are still coping and managing. To date, most of what powers data technology throughout the world is a holdover from the 1970s.

Although disk space and processing speed have greatly increased, the core decisions around relational database design remain. As outlined earlier, we now know that it was those decisions that have made changes expensive and high performance elusive. In addition, changes come with greater risk while reducing the capacity to make data more sharable and connected. The name *relational database* even now seems strange considering the amount of effort, cost, and risk involved to create the relationships within them. These factors as well as the progress of supporting technologies have led industries of all types to consider and implement alternatives to the relational database. In the next section, we explore the options that will better connect and analyze data and help us reach the ultimate goals of improved treatments, advancing cures, and progress in patterns of care.

Introduction of NoSQL databases

The term *NoSQL* stems from SQL, or Structure Query Language, which is the primary language used to manage data in relational database systems. In other words, NoSQL has become shorthand for signifying any system that is not a relational database. Although the first use of the term NoSQL dates from the late 1990s, it was only toward the end of the 2000s that NoSQL database solutions were validated in terms of reliable operational usage.[6] Although some technology professionals have taken it to mean "No To SQL," it should rather be viewed as an alternative, as in "Not Only SQL." With the enormous investment to date in relational systems, it will be many years before they are edged out from their current position as the most widely used type of database.

NoSQL options can be divided into one of four different groups or families: *key-value, column-family, document,* and *graph* databases. Each of these groups was designed and is intended to solve discrete use cases. It should be noted that another group, called *multimodel,* is the confluence of each group, which includes combinations of concepts and features from at least two of the four main groups. However, in the context of healthcare, the most intriguing option of the four groups is the graph database.

Graph databases can offer a blend of simplicity and complexity, offer incredible performance as compared to relational systems, and reduce the risk involved with traditionally difficult changes. Graph databases provide relationships a "first-class" status and consider them the core part of the design. While offering extremely solid performance, complex data is a primary driver for graph database adoption, another reason they offer the same tremendous flexibility that is found in so many other NoSQL options. The *schema-free* nature of most graph database options permits the data model to grow and change without giving up any of the speed advantages or adding significant and costly overhead and risk. We cover the three other options in brief, and then return the focus to how graph databases should be considered the first alternative for relational databases inside healthcare data operations.

Key-value databases

Key-value databases, also referred to as key-value stores, represent data by storing large collections of values and providing a single key for each value. Although the values might be duplicated, the keys will be unique. In addition, a given value for a key might be represented as a set of values as opposed to just a single value.

As shown in Figure 3.2, this data structure allows simple values to be stored and accessed by providing the key-value pair. Using a key-value store for simple models, data architects can reduce the amount of time required to think through more complex data models. However, such a simple model places the burden on the application to understand relationships. Key-value databases are fast but sacrifice other traditional features for the sake of speed.

Columnar databases

The column-family database, modeled after Google's Bigtable, can be described simply as rows of objects that contain columns of related data. As with key-value stores, column-family databases also have key values pairs that represent a row. Figure 3.3 shows a simple example of how a columnar data set might be represented. Columnar databases were designed with very large sets of data in mind and where the structure of the data might not be well known. As with key-value stores, creating and analyzing relationships is not the forte of the systems.

Key	Value
1795969139	Richard
1479743393	Clara
7154042678	Louis
7753708318	Aline
2725848812	Andrew
3229863141	Opal
5470739690	Alvin
6223848281	Linda
9557437033	Donald
3426178398	Nancy

Figure 3.2 Example representation of a key-value database.

ID	Fname	Lname	Created	FavoriteColor
1479743393	Clara	Jordan	2013-07-02	Red
1795969139	Richard	Jordan	2013-07-16	Blue
2725848812	Andrew	Wray	2017-06-14	Black
3229863141	Opal	Jordan	2015-10-12	Purple
3426178398	Nancy	Chiozza	2016-01-14	Red
5470739690	Alvin	Jordan	2017-03-06	Brown
6223848281	Linda	Jordan	2013-09-14	Green
7154042678	Louis	Chiozza	2017-10-29	Blue
7753708318	Aline	Wray	2018-09-30	Blue
9557437033	Donald	Jordan	2018-10-31	Blue

Figure 3.3 Example representation of a columnar database.

Document databases

Document databases represent a collection of "documents." Each document has its own collection of keys and values. In some ways, documents contained within a document database are like rows in a relational database (Figure 3.4). In addition, querying against a unique ID or key is a typical method used to retrieve a document. As with other NoSQL options, document databases were also designed to run fast and scale efficiently with requiring the support of extremely large and specialized hardware. This arbitrary approach to system objects has advantages, but, again, places relationship management in the hands of the data architects and programmers.

Graph databases

In its simplest form, a graph database is a collection of objects that are connected by one or more kinds of relationships. The more commonly used graph databases are also known as *property graphs*. The objects are more commonly referred to as vertices, and the relationships are referred to as edges, as shown in Figure 3.5.

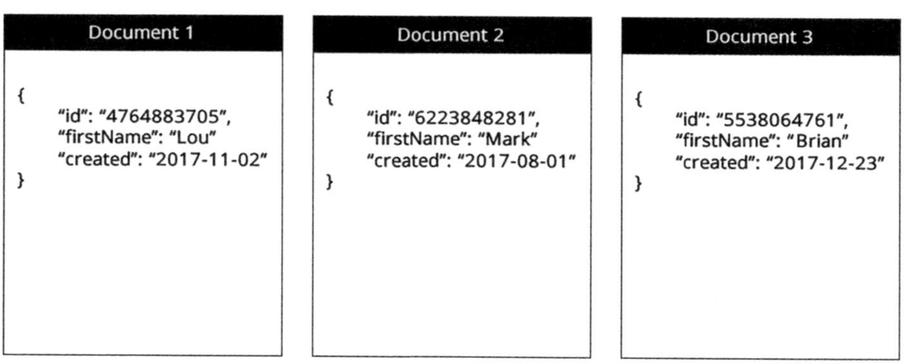

Figure 3.4 Example representation of documents in a document database.

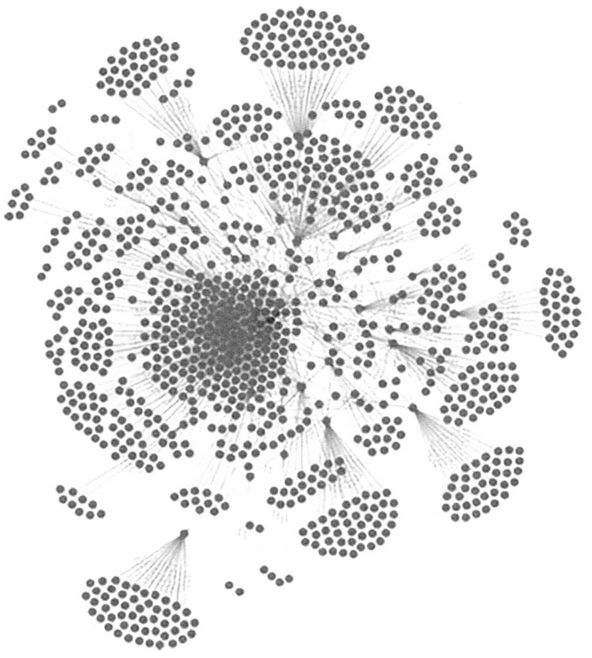

Figure 3.5 Vertices and edges in a graph database.

The terminology as well as the technology are based on graph theory that dates back to the 1700s.[7] Each vertex, like a table name in a relational database or a document in a document database, can assigned a *label*, such as "Patient." Again, like other systems, each vertex can be given keys, such as a name or patient ID, and corresponding values. By grouping vertices in this way, applications can query the graph to show common subsets of what are essentially vertex types. Labeling of vertices also offers a way to enforce modeling constraints when necessary, as well as to increase the speed at which data can be accessed through improved indexing.

While graph databases have some similarities to other systems, the critical difference is that they afford data relationships equal status as compared to other data within the system. As discussed earlier, the schema-free design of graph databases permits data models to change and evolve without sacrificing any of the speed, reduce the risk of problems during changes, as well as allow for changes to occur much more quickly as compared to systems that have rigid schema requirements.

Graph use cases

One of the most well-known use cases for graphs is social networks. The natural way a graph system can create relationships between a person and other things, whether it is people on LinkedIn or people and posts on Facebook, has allowed these organizations to scale to billions of users. Graphs also excel at revealing paths and patterns of data, such as a route to the airport or a product recommendation engine on Amazon. In the field of healthcare data, graphs can offer a new way forward in understanding the impact of the smallest decision.

Referral patterns and patient outcomes

Before a patient can visit with a specialist, it is a common practice to have an initial visit with a primary care physician (PCP). This methodology has origins from the 1800s but has been more formally organized in the past half-century.[8] Two purposes of this methodology are to avoid unnecessary visits as well as help control costs. A PCP can act as a gatekeeper between the patient and more expensive, specialized services. One concern of the methodology is the variability of referral practices of PCPs and the impact it has on patient outcomes.[9]

To that end, there are hundreds of studies that examine the relationship between referral patterns of PCPs and their patients' outcomes. These studies often focus on patterns within a single specialty and use a random sample of patients or physicians. One reason authors and investigators need to narrow their focus on a single specialty can be traced to the structure of the data. These structures of the database and systems are designed for the capture of information as a record and not to operationalize the data for analysis and improvements. Graph databases can remove this constraint. As shown, graphs can display the paths that patients take from their PCPs to the specialty and connected specialists. Finding and analyzing the data and outcomes of patients that take the same path becomes possible over much larger data sets and variable patterns.

As described in *Visualizing Collaborative Electronic Health Record Usage for Hospitalized Patients with Heart Failure*, the investigators sought to monitor care coordination in a "provider collaboration network" by creating a "graph-based analysis method to identify healthcare interactions among populations known to experience high readmission rates."[10] Their first step in that goal was to focus on patients hospitalized with heart failure. As they analyzed the data using a graph, the researchers got a clearer picture of complex interactions between healthcare professionals.

Using a graph, these paths can be more easily visualized and reveal the discrete patterns that lead to favorable and unfavorable patient outcomes. While the patterns alone are not the key to reproducing good outcomes or eliminating bad ones, they do provide a more specific understanding of who, what, and where to further investigate. Finally, as the graph increases in both variety and volume of data, it can be multipurposed to explore the impact beyond each specific specialty and hospital but across specialties and hospital networks.

Medical errors

Reducing the rate of medical errors represents an enormous challenge to healthcare organizations. Martin Makary, professor of surgery at the Johns Hopkins University

School of Medicine, produced a study in 2016 that suggested medical errors were the third leading cause of death in the United States.[11] One common misconception is that medical errors are nearly always the result of a careless or bad healthcare professional.

On the contrary, the errors are usually a result of variability within a network that does not have visibility and, consequently, will not lead to accountability. "Unwarranted variation is endemic in health care. Developing consensus protocols that streamline the delivery of medicine and reduce variability can improve quality and lower costs in health care," says Makary.[12]

Medical errors, like referral patterns, have paths and patterns that can be more readily identified using a graph database. As shown, graph analysis that shows the path that patients take, beginning with their PCPs, could reveal a pattern that has a higher likelihood of resulting in a medical error. The paths can show where variance does and does not occur, which helps healthcare institutions understand where to spend time to best address the problem.

Fraud

For the United States, healthcare spending represents nearly 20% of the gross domestic product.[13] When combined with the volume of encounters and complexity of the system as well as the tens of millions of healthcare employees, healthcare becomes a rich target for fraudulent behavior. Fraud, specifically theft and embezzlement, for a single encounter can be hidden among the dozens of items in an insurance claim. For example, MedStar Ambulance, Inc., agreed to pay $12.7 million to settle a lawsuit that alleged the company knowingly billed Medicare for ambulance trips that were deemed unnecessary.[14] On an annual basis, one estimate states that fraud and abuse cost the healthcare system as much as $272 billion each year.[15] Even reducing fraud and abuse by 1% could have a significant impact on reducing the cost of healthcare.

When searching for fraud using current systems, it is often the case that the fraudulent activity took place well before it was discovered. In *Graph databases for large-scale healthcare systems*, the researchers suggest that graphs can help find the fraud as it occurs rather than after the fact. As with the other use cases, the paths and relationships represent the critical points in the discovery, and the seeming variability of events can be shown as patterns. As the researchers explain, the structure of a graph database fits the network of actors and involved parties and "investigation on these relationships often leads to early detection on organized frauds."[16]

Bring graphs and graph analysis into the organization

There are organizations that offer graph analytical services that address these use cases, but these organizations often approach the data architecture and technology without regard to vertical variability, let alone the variability that can occur from one hospital or physician network to the next. For many healthcare organizations, undertaking these programs internally, even with just a small group focused on it, will ultimately yield greater results and value than outsourcing this analysis. Once the technology has been in place and continually utilized, it is just a matter of time before the knowledge to uncover these patterns becomes an institutional ability. As the expertise grows, this will make it relatively easier to share data outside the organization and better examine and understand referral patterns, reduce medical errors, and combat fraud as a cooperative or collaborative mission.

Summary

These are just a handful of the established use cases where connected data inside healthcare organizations can be applied. As the use of graph databases and new data architecture are increasingly fostered within the healthcare domain, we will begin to see patterns emerge that have higher levels of confidence and quality because they are based on a breadth and depth of data connectivity not possible with legacy systems.

The exponential growth of data combined with keeping systems highly available, accurate, and precise are a daunting prospect. The elements of cost and performance, risk, and data connectivity are the first steps in tackling those larger issues. Technology professionals and administrators should first look to developing and nurturing a culture that explores new data options and alternatives. The most successful organizations will look to reduce their dependency on legacy systems and move toward data architectures and systems, like graph databases, that can more readily and easily make sense of the complex world of healthcare data.

References

1. Digital Universe Driving Data Growth in Healthcare. EMC Digital Universe with Research and Analysis by IDC online, last modified April 2014. https://www.emc.com/analyst-report/digital-universe-healthcare-vertical-report-ar.pdf
2. Barrett, L. Hospital Revives Its 'Dead' Patients, last modified February 10, 2003. http://www.baselinemag.com/c/a/Projects-Networks-and-Storage/Hospital-Revives-Its-QTEDeadQTE-Patients
3. Codd, E. F. June 1970. A relational model of data for large shared data banks. *Communications of the ACM*, 13(6), 377–387.
4. Sewell, J. P., Linda, Q. T. 2013. *Informatics and Nursing: Opportunities and Challenges.* Philadelphia, PA: Wolters Kluwer Health/Lippincott Williams & Wilkins.
5. A History of Storage Cost, last modified September 9, 2009. http://www.mkomo.com/cost-per-gigabyte
6. Vardanyan, M. Picking the Right NoSQL Database Tool, last modified July 6, 2017. http://www.monitis.com/blog/picking-the-right-Nosql-database-tool/
7. Alexanderson, G. L. October 2006. Euler and Konigsberg's bridges: A historical view. *Bulletin of the American Mathematical Society*, 43(4), 567–573.

8. Gutierrez, C., Scheid, P. The History of Family Medicine and Its Impact in US Health Care Delivery, accessed March 15th, 2018. https://www.aafp.org/dam/foundation/documents/who-we-are/cfhm/FMImpactGutierrezScheid.pdf
9. Cowen, M., Zodet, M. August 1999. Methods for analyzing referral patterns. *Journal of General Internal Medicine*, 14(8), 474–480.
10. Soulakis, N. et al. March 2015. Visualizing collaborative electronic health record usage for hospitalized patients with heart failure. *Journal of the American Medical Informatics Association*, 22(2), 299–311.
11. Makary, M. A., Daniel, M. Medical error—The third leading cause of death in the US. *British Medical Journal*, 353, i2139, last modified May 3, 2016. https://www.bmj.com/content/353/bmj.i2139
12. Study Suggests Medical Errors Now Third Leading Cause of Death in the U.S., last modified May 3, 2016. https://www.hopkinsmedicine.org/news/media/releases/study_suggests_medical_errors_now_third_leading_cause_of_death_in_the_us
13. The $272 billion swindle, last modified May 31, 2014. https://www.economist.com/news/united-states/21603078-why-thieves-love-americas-health-care-system-272-billion-swindle
14. $12.7 Million Settlement in Whistleblower Medicare Fraud Case Against Mass. Agency, *EMSWorld* online, last modified January 16, 2017. https://www.emsworld.com/news/12294994/-12-7-million-settlement-in-whistleblower-medicare-fraud-case-against-mass-agency
15. Berwick, D. M., Hackbarth, A. D. April 11, 2012. Eliminating waste in US health care. *Journal of the American Medical Association*, 307(14), 1513–1516.
16. Park, Y. et al. 2014. Graph databases for large-scale healthcare systems: A framework for efficient data management and data services. *2014 IEEE 30th International Conference on Data Engineering Workshops*, 12–19.

Chapter 4

Knowledge management for health data analytics

Charisse Madlock-Brown, Ian M. Brooks, and James Beem

CONTENTS

Each year healthcare becomes even more information intensive, with systems capturing colossal volumes of data daily.[1] In 2012, digital healthcare data was estimated to be equal to 500 petabytes worldwide and is expected to reach 25,000 petabytes in 2020.[2] For reference, a petabyte is 1000 terabytes, or 1,000,000 gigabytes. With this vast and rapid increase in data collection, there have been necessary and concomitant advancements in data processing. Within the healthcare community in the United States, there is great interest in applying advanced analytic tools to improve care, save lives, and lower costs.[3] Data mining, machine learning, and natural language processing seem poised to overhaul the entire healthcare system to usher in an era defined by precision medicine, advanced disease surveillance, reduced errors, and advanced clinical decision support tools. However, applying existing technologies is hampered by data governance and infrastructure issues that impact data quality, systems interoperability, and data alignment.[4] Also, few in the healthcare community are trained in algorithm-based analytics.[5] This chapter focuses first on the necessity of putting data management layers in place before applying more advanced tools is possible. We discuss these processes within the framework of *knowledge management* (KM). KM is the academic discipline that studies and effects the transformation of data into information, and the application of that new information to create actionable knowledge. We discuss the current state of analytics technologies that could then be applied and discuss the impact that it could have on healthcare in the United States.

Rise of the electronic health record

In 2009 the American Recovery and Reinvestment Act (ARRA) was signed into law. As part of the ARRA, the Health Information Technology for Economic and Clinical Health (HITECH) Act was implemented, providing several significant updates to clinical and health privacy law at that point. While many of the provisions of the HITECH Act can be considered as updates to penalty and liability clauses of the Health Insurance Portability and Accountability Act (HIPAA)—designed specifically to increase patient privacy in a more technological word—other clauses are important to our discussion in this chapter. A significant provision of the HITECH Act linked financial incentives and reimbursements from the Centers for Medicare and Medicaid Services (CMS) to the staged adoption of a series of four provisions meant to drive adoption of electronic health records (EHRs) across hospital systems and doctor's offices in the United States. These four provisions are referenced as Meaningful Use (originally four stages, but reduced to three when CMS became a key player). In order to qualify for financial incentives, providers had to meet certain benchmarks in the drive to reduce and eliminate paper-based patient records. The goals were to increase security and privacy protections for patient data; reduce repetitive and needless medical testing by allowing increased data sharing between providers; and begin to move to a more outcomes-based reimbursement system, where providers could be compensated for keeping patients out of hospitals instead of only being paid when patients were sick enough to need emergency or inpatient care.

The launch of the Meaningful Use initiatives created a vibrant marketplace for EHR vendors. No longer were these expensive add-ons for the richest of clinics, but were now mandated and essential tools for modern care. A 2015 report by the Office of the National Coordinator for Health Information Technology demonstrated that in 2009 (when HITECH became law) just under 10% of hospitals had EHRs. By 2015 when the report was published, almost 97% of hospitals had EHRs (https://www.healthit.gov/sites/default/files/data-brief/2014HospitalAdoptionDataBrief.pdf).

It is beyond the remit of this chapter to address the rapid and lightly regulated adoption and the possible effects that may still be observed on hospital expenditures, effects on patient care processes and workflows, and how it affected smaller independent clinics that merged with powerful systems with the offer of a "free" EHR to meet otherwise impossible Meaningful Use targets. What we cannot deny, however, is this growth -period of EHR adoption has led to the creation of new powerful technologies, creation of vast data resources, driven massive surges in medical clinical research, and development of new data and software standards.

For the purposes of this chapter, the excitement and potential of such vast data resources are tempered by the complexity of the rules surrounding interinstitutional data sharing, and the lack of interoperability between EHR systems, even those provided by the same vendor. We are faced now with great potential for healthcare research and the opportunity to conduct truly population scale clinical research. We have rich data assets, and now must focus our interests on developing the tools, training, procedures, and workflows to help create the skilled labor force we will need in the years ahead.

Data governance and infrastructure issues

As healthcare reform sets new standards and evaluation metrics for healthcare systems, complex systems integration and data integrity are required to keep hospitals up to date with accountable healthcare. Establishing a culture of value measurement in healthcare, as in any other industry, involves developing a shared understanding of how the value of data is defined so it can be measured, analyzed, managed, and monitored. A cross-functional data governance model will help healthcare organizations (HCOs) harness value from their stored information. It is essential that a chain of trust is created so both the producers and the consumers of the data are confident it is appropriately used and accurate for its purpose. The wealth of data collected across an enterprise needs to be appropriately, consistently, and accurately brought together—integrated—to provide timely and reliable information. The data chain of trust from source to integration needs to be clear and well documented, at which point the resulting integrated view can then be considered the source of truth for information to support the reporting, measurement, and analytics needs of an organization. To be clear, data governance is not an information technology (IT) function, or a department in the organizational hierarchy. Rather, it is a process that sets standards for capturing and transferring data across systems. It institutes decisions about how to resolve inconsistencies and dictates access, security, and patient privacy.

According to the Data Governance Institute, "data governance is a system of decision rights and accountabilities for information-related processes, executed according to agreed-upon models which describe who can take what actions with what information, and when, under what circumstances, using what methods."[6] This definition emphasizes the protocols that determine the access rights and business rules that determine information processes. Though this definition is relevant for healthcare, it is limited. An alternative from TechTarget states that it is "the overall management of the availability, usability, integrity, and security of data used in an enterprise."[7] This second definition explicitly states the types of issues governances is meant to resolve. Particularly relevant for healthcare is the issue of integrity, which refers to the quality of data. Good data governance is largely missing in healthcare. In 2014, the American Health Information Management Association (AHIMA) conducted a survey on information governance in healthcare, which revealed that 35% of 1,000 healthcare respondents did not know if their organization had any information governance efforts underway, or did not recognize a need for a governance program.[8]

Good data governance allows hospitals to set policies in place which dictate rules on allowable data values and data types. These processes can help those institutions avoid errors and reduce duplications in data collection. These changes are reflected indirectly through more effective use of employee time and staffing management, and can have significant financial impacts to an enterprise organization by increasing efficiencies and reducing costly errors. As we discuss, the back-end systems managing our vast reservoirs of medical and health data are distributed and complex. Proper data governance ensures stored information about patients is correct; the system captures the right information and timely access to data for analytics purposes and reporting. More indirect effects can be seen when we consider the ability to reuse and share properly managed resources across an enterprise. Access to and use of medical data are protected by HIPAA. In the Code of Federal Regulations chapter 46 (46 CFR 164.502(b)), we are reminded to always use the minimal necessary standard when working with patient data (https://www.hhs.gov/hipaa/for-professionals/index.html). Although usually considered a guideline rather than an enforced rule, it behooves us to remember to respect our patients' privacy at all times, which can be effected by not needlessly duplicating data for duplicate reports or key performance metrics.

Data governance can greatly affect analysis and reporting. One of the most significant issues affecting the translation of clinical research to improved population care is replication and reproducibility.[9] The number and variety of data sources for clinical studies have increased 10-fold in the last decade. When reproducibility is in question, accurate metadata can help answer questions concerning data generation, data definitions, and data transformations. For instance, it is common to discover duplicate patient records in a large data set if all participants have not been derived from a single system. Analysts need stringent data governance and data design models. Connections such as deletion, merging, and imputation of missing variables must also be recorded in the metadata layer.

Absent data governance, the likelihood that any technology introduced into an HCO will succeed is small. Organizations must be confident that the data represented within the technology are reliable and accurate—data governance provides the structure and process to ensure the needed reliability and accuracy. Without data governance, the implemented technology may function exactly as designed, but the information emanating from the technology may be suspect.

Health information exchange infrastructure

Today, most HCOs lack access to data from across the continuum of care, because their EHRs are not interoperable with those of other providers and HCOs. Though some EHR vendors have committed to addressing this issue, today the information in these disparate EHRs cannot be exchanged in a form that clinicians and researchers can review and act on. While progress has been made in exchanging standardized care summaries between different EHRs, these summaries are in the form of documents, not discrete data.

The Office of the National Coordinator for Health Information Technology (ONC) defines interoperability as "the ability of a system to exchange electronic health information from other systems without special effort on the part of the user."[10] This has long been a key goal of healthcare leaders and policy experts, who say that interoperability is a prerequisite for obtaining true value from IT systems. In its 2017 interoperability roadmap, however, ONC acknowledges that interoperability has not yet arrived. A recent survey of healthcare executives, similarly, found only 8% of providers had interoperability with other providers and were integrating outside data into their workflow.[11] Consequently, most of the health information exchange (HIE) that occurs today is confined to sending and receiving documents, such as care summaries. These documents are generally transmitted in the Consolidated Clinical Data Architecture (CCDA) format. Direct secure messaging, which can be used to convey these care summaries, is increasingly popular and may be embedded in some EHR systems, but it is still not widespread. Record locators are increasingly being used to retrieve documents from distributed databases.

A database designed for healthcare management typically must manage two major types of data: administrative/billing data and diagnostic/medical data. Although these two data sets are describing the same patient, the information they reveal can have subtle and surprising differences. It is beyond the scope of this chapter to discuss in detail all of these differences, but suffice it to say, what your physician codes you for when you have an encounter (via *International Classification of Diseases* [*ICD*] and *Current Procedural Terminology* [*CPT*] codes, for example) is not always what is reported back via your billing data. Additionally, because of the time lags in financial reconciliation, there can be discrepancies between dates. These differences are subtle but can have powerful confounding effects to clinical and quality improvement questions. Claims data, which provides a very broad view of a patient's care, can also be integrated with clinical data. But it requires considerable technical expertise to parse claims information, and great care must be taken when combining it with clinical data. For example, when a provider orders a test to rule out a diagnosis, that does not mean that the patient has that diagnosis, yet a code for it may appear on a claim for the test. Claims must be compared with clinical data to eliminate these kinds of errors. To resolve these issues, developers created three different network models to deal with transferring data between systems.[12]

The first type of model is the centralized model, which is also known as an HIE. The HIE connects payer, provider, and public health data sources through a single common data pool. In some states these are run by state-level organizations, for example, the Chesapeake Regional Information System for our Patients (CRISP) in Maryland, which was founded by a like-minded group of hospital chief information officers in 2006 and formalized as the nonprofit Maryland HIE. Other HIEs are more organic, created by like-minded local groupings of hospitals and providers responding to a state or federal mandate, for example, the MidSouth eHealth Alliance (MSeHA), in Memphis, Tennessee.

Within an HIE, organizations transfer information into an aggregated clinical data repository. This type is simple and highly effective for aggregating information from multiple sources, and works well for community-level data analytics, population health management, and financial analyses. However, the complexity and scale of data provide for some limitations, such as providers being more likely to receive static reports rather than be able to perform analytics on the fly. Funding restrictions may also lead to technical limitations on what might be done with data or user interfaces. Given the scale and profound and obvious risk undergirding HIE databases, they invariably require strong central coordination and very strict data governance methods. Data submission for participating systems may lag, and it is likely to be a fairly expensive option to implement. Nevertheless, an well-managed HIE can provide incredible resources for healthcare providers and hospital system financial and operations leadership who are users of a single HIE vendor.

A second and converse method of data management at scale is the federated, or decentralized, model. In a federated model, data remain at their source and are queried using a distributed search method—a central point receives the query and sends it out to each member who then reports their data back. These separate reports are then combined and presented to the user. In some cases, this distributed query may be managed by software; in others, a safe harbor and honest broker provide the service. A federated model gives healthcare providers control over their patient information. Participants agree on data access, which removes the question of data ownership. This model prevents many problems with privacy and security that may arise when keeping data in one large pool. Importantly, it offers a defense against single-point failure where one member may bring down an organization's data structure during a technical difficulty. However, because providers can maintain more control over their data, issues of data sharing and access protocols to local systems can derail negotiations. Because data is not stored by an HIE system, data controls are not guaranteed, and standards definitions can be hard to define and enforce, meaning customized reports need to be developed for each query and participating system.

In an attempt to resolve the issues associated with the HIE/central and federated model systems, hybrid models were developed. Hybrids are a cross between both systems, hopefully combining the best and minimizing the worst of features. This model provides an interface engine for which organizational entities in the HIE communicate. The Tennessee eHealth Volunteer Initiative uses a model in which data is physically stored and managed in a central location, but the data is logically separated into volumes managed by each organization that contributes data. In this model, key record identifiers are stored and used to gather and transfer medical information, and only some of the data is stored centrally.

An important component of all of these models, in addition to the data governance described previously, is the integration engine needed to connect multiple systems using standard protocols. The integration engine may perform many tasks and typically uses messaging protocols like HL7 to provide many of the functions to ensure storage of the right data in the right place. Another vital task is patient-matching. Can we confirm that the patient with the same name in one database is the same as in another? Or should they be two separate records? What about common name variations and misspellings? We cannot use Social Security number as a reliable marker, and the United States does not provide patients with a unique identifier used across medical systems. In fact, HIPAA regulations required the development of a proposed rule for national patient identities, but public opposition to providing the ability for an entity to track all medical information for patients has defeated its development. Therefore, the integration engine must use multiple points of patient information, such as gender, date of birth, telephone number, etc., to drive an algorithm that statistically matches patients across and between data sets. This is not an ideal situation and can have profound effects when studying orphan (rare) diseases or working with medically underserved communities, such as minorities, and patients who are at high risk for substance abuse, self-harm, and homelessness, such as transgender people, and military veterans, as well as other at-risk groups.

Following, we discuss these and other models in more depth. We do not subscribe to the theory that "one size fits all" when managing enterprise-scale data resources. Rather, leadership must make informed decisions regarding which solution or solutions will provide the most valuable knowledge management environment, bearing in mind that multiple solutions of various scales may be necessary to reach all intended goals and use cases.

Health information exchange

Compared to even just a few years ago, today's research questions are often dauntingly complex, a characteristic reflected in the data required for such research. Data are often needed from multiple data sources, including laboratory values, unstructured text records of clinical findings (recorded clinical notes), cost and quality information, and genetic data. In addition, research on less common clinical conditions—those with low incidence or prevalence—inherently demands larger data sets with greater geographic and demographic diversity. Data from a single organization are often insufficient for many research questions aimed at gaining the depth of understanding required to support evidence-based practices tailored to individuals. Thus, there is a growing need for data sharing across research entities and collaborators. Sharing data across computer systems is often a perilous journey, with possible distortions and uncertain arrivals. The ability of EHRs to integrate with outside applications designed for population health management is difficult. As with EHR-to-EHR data exchange, the proprietary code underlying EHRs prevents them from linking to applications without special interfaces.

HIE is an emerging format with the potential to greatly facilitate improvements in healthcare quality, efficiency, and data interoperability.[13] Data governance models achieve these improvements. The Healthcare Information and Management Systems Society (HIMSS) defines an HIE as a system that "automates the transfer of health-related information that is typically stored in multiple organizations while maintaining the context and integrity of the infoımation being exchanged."[14] These systems rely on data value standards to deal with interoperability issues across hospital systems. These systems are used to integrate data between similar systems and also across disparate systems. Currently, in the United States, there is not a single-source information management system that can facilitate all administrative, clinical, and laboratory tasks for large healthcare systems. This means the IT background and infrastructure undergirding any healthcare enterprise is complex, and sometimes highly so. Managing the layers of integration necessary for hospital operations (finance and operations, supply chain management), quality (patient safety), and clinical research can mean adding infrastructural complexity while attempting to increase interoperability, which means adding more layers of independent vendor products and software. There are numerous health information technology (HIT) systems, such as electronic medical records systems, radiology information systems, laboratory information systems, pharmacy information systems, and pediatric health information systems. Data from medical devices, such as pumps and patient monitoring systems, and diagnostic and treatment devices also generate information that needs to be integrated for analysis, data sharing, and patient profiling.

An effective HIE addresses issues related to the six dimensions of interoperability, the four levels of interoperability, and the four standards categories, as follows.[14]

The six dimensions of interoperability are

- Uniform movement of healthcare data
- Uniform presentation of data
- Uniform user interface controls
- Uniform safeguarding of data security and integrity
- Uniform protection of confidentiality
- Uniform assurance of common degree of system service quality

The four levels of interoperability are

- Nonelectronic information (such as paper records)
- Machine-transportable information (electronic nonstandardized data)
- Machine-organizable information (structured but nonstandardized and uses an interface for communication between two or more systems)
- Machine-interpretable information (standardized and coded data such as patient diagnosis data using *ICD-10* codes)

The four standards categories are

- Transport standards (address exchanged message formats)
- Content standards (define the structure and content of the electronic message)
- Vocab standard (represent health concepts in an encoded structured way)
- Security standards (define safeguards that protect the privacy and security of health information)

These classifications aid providers in planning and selecting the type and level of interoperability required to achieve successful HIE. Each interoperability issue must classify issues by standards type. Hospital systems can achieve these by reviewing high-level HIT standards documentation. An example of HIE success was establishing interoperability between vital records (VRs) and her, which resulted in more timely data release, and higher-quality data for demographic and epidemiologic surveillance and research. It also led to less costly electronic vital registration systems, greater integration with other stakeholder systems, and greater standardization of VR data collection and exchange.[15]

To accomplish effective HIE, providers must choose an interoperability standard. The HL7 v2.x suite is one of the most widely used standards in the world for communicating clinical data among clinical information systems.[16] It provides specifications for messaging to support information sharing, admission, transfer, and discharge. The HL7 v3 suite increased the detail, clarity, and precision of message specification (Figure 4.1).

Disease registries

A significant role can be played by informaticians in the development, creation, and maintenance of disease registries. In its most basic form, a disease registry is a data mart combining data extracted from one or more sources from a foundation query built around a specific disease diagnosis and/or treatment code. For example, one might be interested in a sole source of truth about all patients with type 2 diabetes within a population, or those with breast cancer diagnoses. Disease registries are powerful tools for healthcare research; well-designed registries can have broad utility in patient recruiting, patient outcomes, patient safety, quality of care, financial reimbursement, and provider incentives, and also play auxiliary roles (in combination with other sources) in supply chain management and product development. However, before building a disease registry, it is worth the investment of time of multiple stakeholders to define the purpose and proposed end-state of the product. If the underlying data structure is in the form of a well-maintained relational database, then having "too much" data is merely a question of governance and privacy. But if running a registry based on a flat-file format (such as a spreadsheet-based system), then increasing the number of variables will slow read-in and readout times, as well as lead to inefficient and slower data analysis.

Increasing recognition is being given to the real-world informatics and IT challenges that underlie such seemingly simple tools. More hospital and other networks are now creating enhanced registries that make use of data governance models to ensure valid data is created for analysis and monitoring.[17] Given the complexity inherent in expecting multiple, disparate data systems (e.g. EHRs) to communicate, a vital data governance task is ensuring that meaning is consistent and transferable across systems. To this end, developers need data dictionaries to guarantee legal values for data types and provide precise definitions for

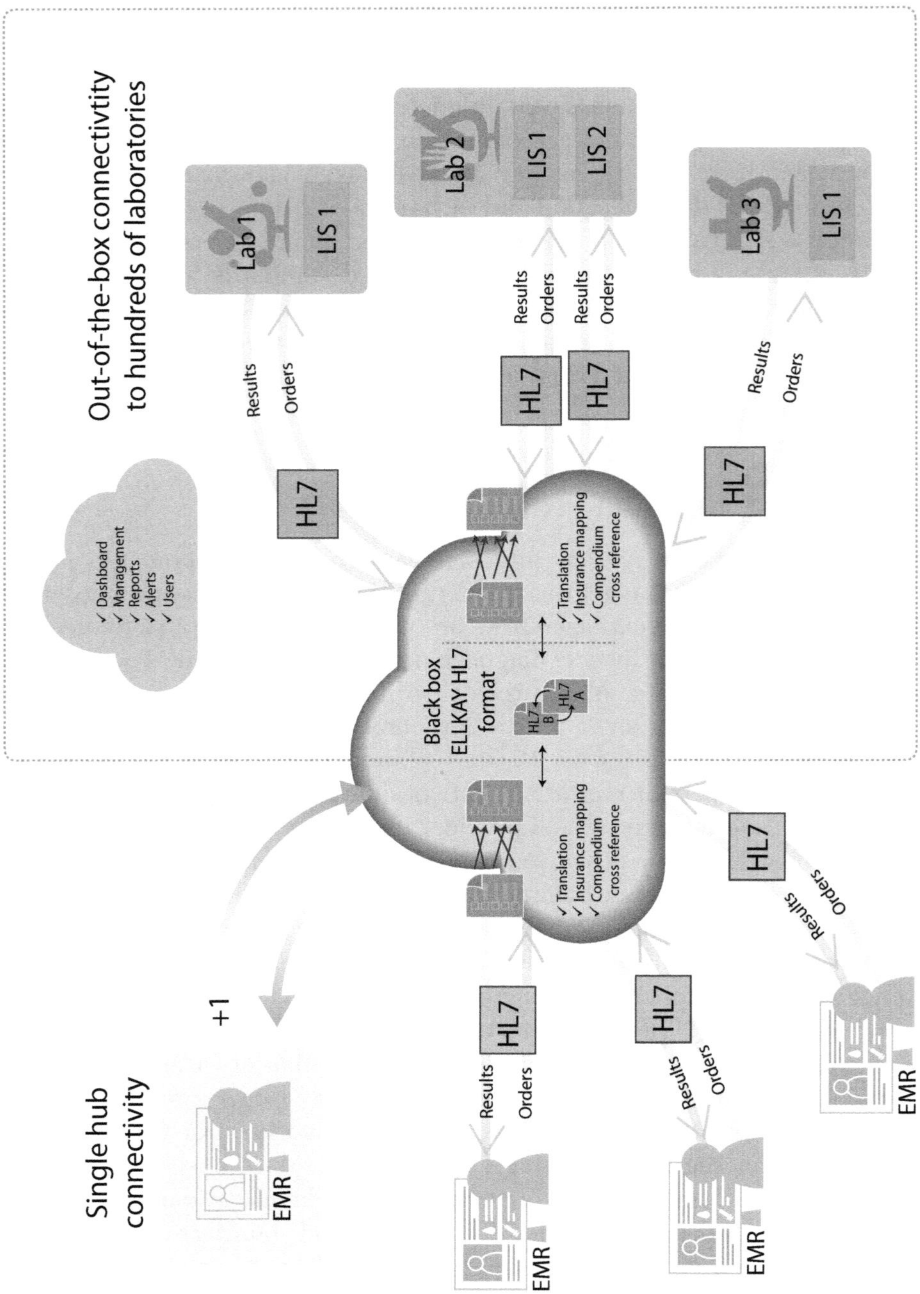

Figure 4.1 HIE using HL7.

terminology. Again, the input of a variety of stakeholders is essential in ensuring that interoperability is true at the "semantic" level (the implied meaning of a variable), as well as at a more obvious "syntactic" level (the underlying fact of a variable). Standardization and creation of common data models (CDMs) have greatly aided this effort. Common data elements (CDEs) were created by the National Cancer Institute to address the need for consistent cancer research terminology.

Although disease registries can have great utility, we must remember that the complexity of modern healthcare data-space usually precludes a "one-size-fits-all" approach. While remembering the tenets of HIPAA and good data governance and avoiding needless duplication of data or effort, we must also consider other models that might fit larger enterprise needs. In addressing these, we move away from the traditional database scale, and permanence of thought that drives a disease registry initiative, into the larger space of the data warehouse, and the flexibility of the data lake.

Data warehouses and data lakes

There are very few published articles on data warehouse governance for healthcare systems. James Walker defined data warehouse governance as "the model the organization will use to ensure optimal use and re-use of the data warehouse and enforcement of corporate policies and ultimately derive value for the money." [18] Data warehouse governances require a focus on ensuring security, privacy, and regulatory compliance, as well as data provenance.

The vast majority of HCOs now use enterprise data warehouses (EDWs) to aggregate and analyze their own data. But their ability to do so is largely dependent on their size. In a recent survey, 94% of hospitals with 200 or fewer beds said they were not adequately capturing the data they needed for population health management analytics.[19]

As government-mandated healthcare regulatory requirements and the need for enterprise-wide data analysis continue to grow, many companies and large government entities are looking to attain standard definitions for their common data within the EDW environment. Not surprisingly, these same organizations have come to the realization that a managed metadata environment is necessary to persistently store and technically manage those definitions; however, it is only half of the equation. There is also a business side to defining the processes and procedures necessary to initially create and manage these common data definitions on an ongoing basis. These processes and procedures are known as data governance and stewardship.

HCOs frequently customize their EHRs to meet their needs and goals. As a result, the data mapping performed on their behalf can quickly become outdated. Naturally, this is much more complicated when several different data sources are involved. Moreover, the public and private payers that seek quality data from healthcare providers often change their measures, and HCOs may pick different metrics from one year to the next. When this happens, different kinds of data must be integrated to produce quality reports. To ensure that these changes do not reduce the accuracy of data mapping, the data must be remapped at regular intervals or as needed.

Given the complexity and cost of traditional data warehouses, many organizations can use *data lakes* to expedite the process.[20] A data lake is an easily scalable, accessible data repository of raw data in its native format. Data is transformed when needed, and big data analytics solutions can be integrated. Though data lakes are potentially reasonable solutions to large-scale data management needs, lack of inherent governance is their biggest drawback. A data lake should be managed with a life-cycle management tool so developers can take advantage of their scalability and low cost (see Figure 4.2).

Dimension	Enterprise data warehouse	Data lake
Workload	Hundreds to thousands of concurrent users performing interactive analytics using advanced workload management capabilities to enhance query performance. Batch processing	Batch processing of data at scale. Currently improving its capabilities to support more interactive users
Schema	Typically schema is defined before data is stored. Schema on write means required data is identified and modeled in advance. Requires work at the beginning of the process, but offers performance, security, and integration . Works well for data types where data value is known	Typically schema is defined after data is stored. Schema on read means data must be captured in code for each program accessing the data. Offers extreme agility and ease of data capture, but requires work at the end of the process. Works well for data types where data value is not known
Scale	Can scale to large data volumes at moderate cost	Can scale to extreme data volumes at low cost
Access methods	Data accessed through standard SQL and standardized B1 tools, which are supported by many different systems for reporting and analytics	Data accessed through programs created by developers. SQL-like systems, and other methods
Benefits	Very fast response times Consistent performance High concurrency Easy to consume data Rationalization of data from multiple sources into a single enterprise view Clean, safe, secure data Cross-functional analysis Transform once, use many	Executes on tens to thousands of servers with superb scalability Parallelization of traditional programming languages (Java, C++, Python, Perl, etc.) Supports higher level programming frameworks such as Pig and HiveQL Radically changes the economic model for storing high volumes of data
SQL	ANSI SQL , ACID compliant	Flexible programming, evolving SQL
Data	Cleansed	Raw
Access	Seeks	Scans
Complexity	Complex joins	Complex processing
Cost/Efficiency	Efficient use of CPU/IO	Low cost of storage and processing

Figure 4.2 Comparing the enterprise data warehouse and the data lake.

Following are example use cases:

- The state of Mississippi designed a data lake architecture to collect, store, maintain, and analyze data from a variety of sources in an effort to improve access to care and population management. Currently, many policy makers throughout the state benefit from this application.[21]
- The Georges Popidou University Hospital created a clinical data warehouse (CDW) using i2b2 (information for integrating biology and the bedside) for clinical and epidemiological research. The system contains more than a decade's worth of data for over 860,000 patients. Data was represented using multiple terminologies. The CDW generated multiple secondary data marts used for over 74 different research projects.[22]

Database design issues: Common data models

Although database design tools have been around for decades, many systems are poorly formulated without proper data modeling to reduce data anomalies associated with redundancy, missing data, deletion errors, and incorrect data entry. Further, the companies that develop healthcare databases do not always believe it is in their best interest to create systems that can easily integrate with competitors.

Among the promising solutions to mitigate issues with poorly designed systems are CDMs.[23] CDMs use a standardized schematic for representing structured data such that it reduces data anomalies, reduces redundancy, and supports data integration. They provide a platform-independent relational model, are patient centric, are domain based, and integrate controlled vocabulary for consistent data value. These aspects allow them to uniformly integrate heterogeneous data sources, including registries, claims, and EHR data. Typical data that may not be in a standardized format includes lab results, allergies, immunizations, and health maintenance histories. Except for lab results, the other data types may have custom workflows that vary from one EHR to another. In addition, roughly 60% of the data in an EHR is unstructured, including free text, documents, and images.[24] Medical observations may be dictated by doctors and found in transcribed notes or in documents received from outside sources, such as consultations reports and discharge summaries.

CDMs are extendable and support analytics. These models are developed concerning user needs and common hospital processes and data capture needs. The different systems will then have the same tables, fields, data types, and data dictionaries across different systems. Thereby, dates, conditions, scales, etc., can be perfectly aligned across different systems. For instance, there is a standardization of visit encounters with the basic information captured and stored. Vocabularies support analysis as they can allow researchers to match patients based on medication, disease, and demographics. Different levels of precision are resolved using the vocabulary's concept hierarchy.

Storing data in a CDM is achieved through the extract, transform, and load (ETL) process. ETL moves data from various sources into a data warehouse through the use of a predefined process. This process maps data into the CDM for analysis and storage in the data warehouse. This predefined process must be established concerning organizational requirements, compliance, data profiling, security, integration, right data and right time, and end user interface. When using CDMs, ETL functions can be automated with a database management system and a programming language. The stages are as follows:

1. In the extract phase, data is gathered and cleansed, duplicate or fragmented data is eliminated, and unnecessary data is excluded.
2. In the transform phase, data is prepared for the warehouse, converted using rules and lookup tables, combined when necessary, verified, and finally standardized.
3. In the load phase, transformed data is stored. Batch/real-time processing must be set up. A semantic layer is maintained for future analysis.

The following are example use cases:

- Overhage et al. used the OMOP CDM to integrate data from 10 observational healthcare databases and was able to achieve acceptable data representation using standardized terminologies and perform a wide range of analytic applications.[25]
- Reisinger et al. developed and evaluated a CDM for drug safety surveillance using two types of databases, administrative claims, and electronic medical record databases.[26] Forty-three million patients with approximately 1 billion drug exposures and 3.7 billion condition occurrences from both databases were included in the CDM database. The integrated system produced comparable stored data.

Big data issues

As warehouses, data lakes, and HIE systems store more and more data, the task of processing that data can potentially exceed current technological capabilities regarding storage systems and available memory. Big Data technologies are constantly evolving to deal with these issues. The thresholds for what constitutes big data changes as storage and memory capacity of available machines change. As healthcare information production increases, analysts will need to employ big data solutions.

Commonly referred to as the four Vs, the following characteristics determine the need for big data solutions[27]:

- Value Veracity (ensuring that the data values can be trusted is difficult when data sets are large)
- Velocity (management of data streams when updates are frequent)

- Variety (managing data from a wide variety of applications in a variety of formats)
- Volume (managing data so big that either storing it or processing it on a single machine is nonoptional)

Many HCOs are still in the early phases of developing the competencies that will allow them to achieve the goals of harnessing the valuable data that has been amassed by electronic medical records, operational activities, and transactional systems. Generating actionable insights that can be applied to real-world medical problems is a complicated and challenging task. Introduced by Gartner in 2001, the terms for the mass proliferation of data were coined—volume, velocity, and variety. As enterprises started to collect more types of data, some of which were incomplete or poorly architected, IBM was instrumental in adding the fourth V, veracity, to the mix. The reach of technological innovation continues to grow, changing all industries as it evolves. In healthcare, technology is increasingly playing a role in almost all processes and evolving at a rapid pace. Advanced technologies, such as artificial intelligence, machine learning, and natural language processing, are being marketed throughout the healthcare industry as solutions toward developing insights from healthcare data. However, the reality for HCOs to explore the possibilities of deploying advanced technologies, such as artificial intelligence, will only be realistic after addressing the foundational hurdles that lie below the data challenges of volume, velocity, variety, and veracity. The distribution of clinical data across the health system is highly fragmented, presenting significant challenges in the coordination and aggregation of data resources. To apply the promises of advanced technologies, which are prominent in the conversation today regarding healthcare, it will be equally important to explore strategies to enhance interoperability, address policy, create data standardization, and ensure capability for future data utilities.

Dealing with the issue of veracity takes precise and thoughtful data governance initiatives. Technologies such as HIEs and CDMs can handle issues related to variety.

The following technologies deal with issues of velocity and volume:

- *NoSQL*: A model for distributed database querying and storage[28]
- *Hadoop*: A tool for distributed data processing and management[29]
- *Spark*: An efficient set of libraries with a suite of statistical and data mining tools configured for distributed data processing and management[30]

Importance of data governance and infrastructure

Proper data governance and infrastructure management create a reliable layer on which analytics can be performed. Without it, data cannot necessarily be trusted, accessed, secured, or integrated.

Analytics beyond statistics

Health organizations today are capable of generating and collecting a large amount of data. This increase in data volume automatically requires the data to be retrieved when needed. With the use of data mining techniques, it is possible to extract the knowledge and determine interesting and useful patterns. The knowledge it gained in this way can be used in the proper order to improve work efficiency and enhance the quality of decision-making. Above the foregoing is a great need for new generation of theories and computational tools to help people with extracting useful information from the growing volume of digital data.[31] Information technologies are implemented increasingly often in healthcare organizations to meet the needs of physicians in their daily decision-making. Computer systems used in data mining can be very useful to control human limitations, such as subjectivity and error due to fatigue, and to provide guidance to decision-making processes.[32] The essence of data mining is to identify relationships, patterns, and models that support predictions and decision-making processes for diagnosis and treatment planning. Obtaining information using computers can enhance the quality of decision-making and avoid human error. When there is a large volume of data that must be processed by humans, decision-making is generally of poorer quality.

Data mining is the process of analyzing the raw data using a computer and extracting the meaning of the data. The process is often defined as the discovery of previously unknown and potentially useful information from large volumes of data (unstructured) (Figure 4.3).[33]

Feature selection

Understanding the cause of and trends for many diseases requires the analysis of many features. Environmental, genetic, and lifestyle factors can all contribute to the progression and development of the disease. Selecting features for analysis from high-dimensional data sources to predict disease can be very difficult.[34] The presence of unstructured data, imprecise diagnosis, and lack of interoperability between systems means feature gathering is difficult. Developers must have a clear understanding of the meaning of captured data.

One of the biggest problems in data mining in medicine is that the raw medical data is voluminous and heterogeneous. These data can be gathered from various sources, such as from conversations with patients, laboratory results, review, and interpretation of doctors. All of these components can have a major impact on diagnosis, prognosis, and treatment of the patient, and should not be ignored. Missing, incorrect, inconsistent, or nonstandard data, such as pieces of information saved in different formats from different data sources, create a major obstacle to successful data mining. This is one of the many reasons data governance is essential for the proper application of data mining technologies.

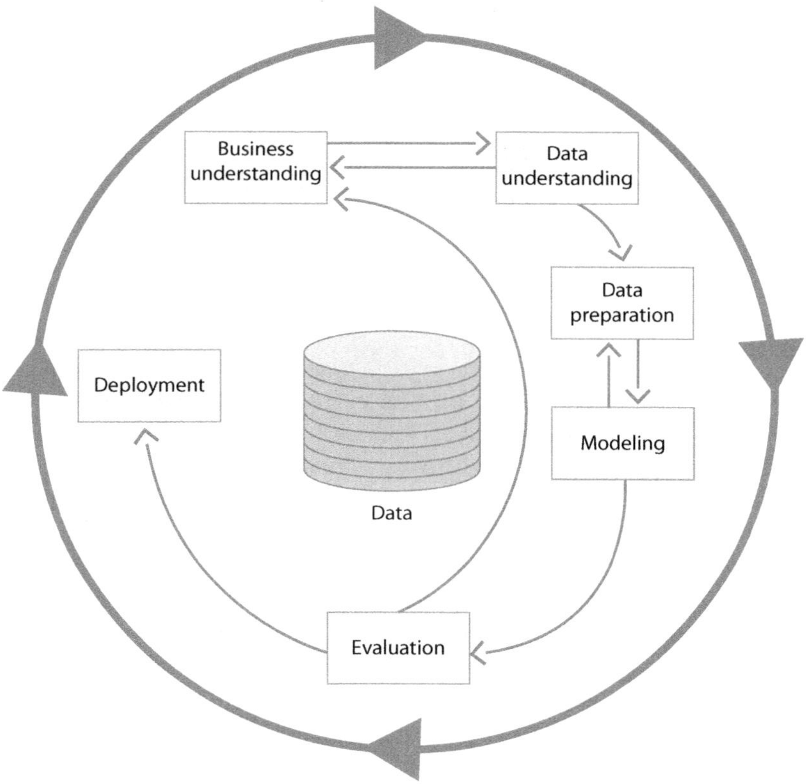

Figure 4.3 Data mining process.

Data is not always gathered for analytics. Therefore, when users want to analyze the data, they need to be very careful about feature selection. When selecting data for analysis, relevant questions may be as follows:

- Relevant and useful information that is stored in the data repository
- Not relevant or useful, and stored in the database

With numerous data fields in healthcare systems, the task of trying to figure out if data is useful may seem daunting. Feature selection algorithms can automate this task. There are two main types of algorithms for this task.[35] The first is *filters*. These procedures order features on possible rankings such as correlation, standard deviation, information gain, missing values, or extreme values. The second type is *wrappers*. These identify the best subset of features by analyzing the various possible permutations of the feature set. This one is very expensive computationally, as the system will need to analyze $(n/k) = n!/k!(n\text{-}k)!$ permutations, where n is number of features and k is the max number of features in a combination.

An example use includes the following:

- The difficulty associated with finding the right features in high-dimensional clinical data repositories impedes the application of analytics solutions. Cheng et al. empirically evaluated the benefits of expert feature selection against automated feature selection. Their results showed that while experts tend to improve the sensitivity of a classifier, the automatic method improves the specificity.[36]

Data mining

The purpose of data mining is to predict accurately in real time or cluster data points, even if that means the analysis lacks interpretability. Parameters are often not interpreted, and the final algorithm is a "black box." Data mining differs from statistics in that statistics attempts to describe the world and the mechanism and variables that contribute to specific outcomes. For statistics, parameters have real-world meaning, confidence intervals are used to capture the variability of the uncertainty of parameters, and assumptions are made about the underlying processes and distributions of the data. Data mining technologies are designed for prediction accuracy and may not give users a sense of the underlying processes that contribute to disease.

You need data mining when you want to predict in real time. For instance, you may want a mechanism that will indicate who might be at risk for diabetes, even if the system cannot tell you why. Also, if you have high dimensionality in your data set and want to perform patient profiling, you may want a process that can deal with potentially dozens of features at once.

Supervised learning

Supervised learning is a technique to use when you are trying to build a model to predict something.[37] The target variable, what you want to predict, must be labeled in your data set. For instance, if you want to predict who will likely have diabetes, you need to have each row of your data labeled with either a "has diabetes" label or a "does not have diabetes" label. The system then builds a model to predict whether new, unlabeled instances should receive the label "has diabetes" or "does not have diabetes." An example of a supervised learning algorithm is a decision tree. One of the main advantages of decision trees is that they are often interpretable. (These are fairly easy to describe and are often used in healthcare.)

Decision trees use the notions of entropy and information to build a tree to predict.[38] The algorithm determines which attributes in a given data set are the most useful in discriminating between the target labels. Entropy is a measurement of disorder. Its equation is $Sum_i - p_i log_2 p_i$, where p_i is the probability of class i. It ranges from 0 to 1 (see Figure 4.4). Information gain measures the entropy you

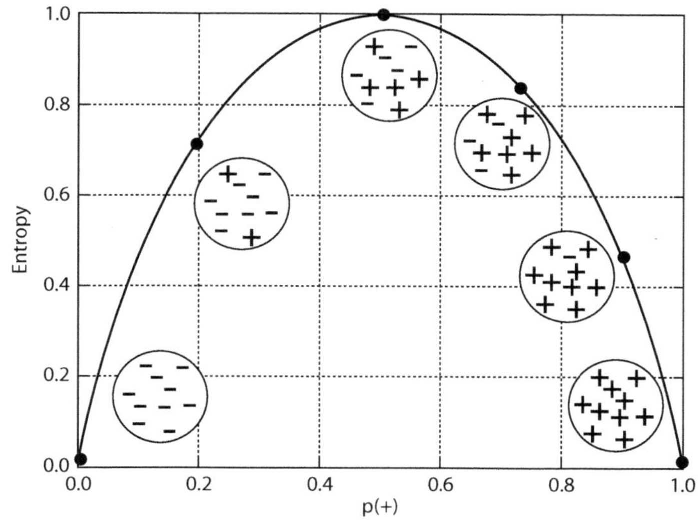

Figure 4.4 Represents relationship between the probability of the positive target label and entropy.

lose if you know the values for an attribute. It is calculated as follows: Entropy (parent) – $Sum_i\ P_i \times entropy_i$, where $entropy_i$ is the entropy of child node i. Each feature will produce two or more child nodes. Decision tree algorithms build a tree where each node splits on the feature with the maximum information gain. It repeats the process for each child node. Information gain is used because considering every possible tree is infeasible. The resultant tree may not be optimal (Figures 4.4 and 4.5).

Supervised learning tools can also be used for decision support tools and to produce a more targeted research and development pipeline in the development of drugs and devices.[39]

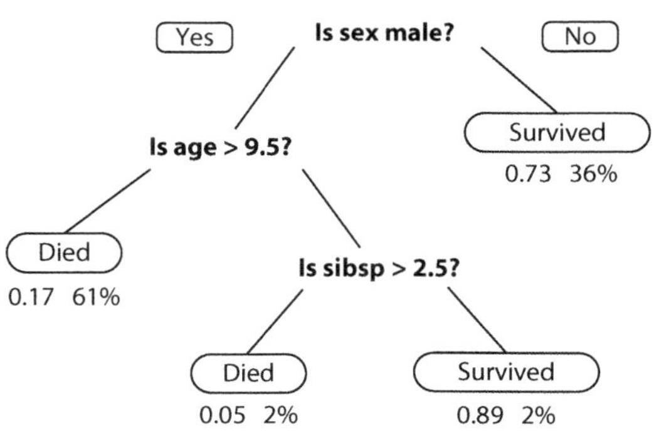

Figure 4.5 Example decision tree from the titanic data set. Commons image.

Following are example use cases:

- Anbarasi et al. used supervised learning classifiers to predict heart disease with 99% accuracy in both "has heart disease" and "does not have heart disease" categories.[40] Their work can help doctors select patients for diagnostic testing.
- Srinivas et al. demonstrated that the use of supervised learning algorithms can not only help predict heart attacks but can also help providers discover new relationships between heart disease and medical factors.[41]

Unsupervised learning

Unsupervised learning is another data mining technique that can be used to segment patient populations. It can be used when you have a large data set with many features, and you want to use those features to group the data.[42] Cluster analysis can be used for analyzing patient characteristics. This is useful for comparative effectiveness research, and disease surveillance, early stage disease prevention, patient recruitment, matching treatment to individuals, and general population health.[43]

Integrated care organizations are moving beyond just delivering care to patients toward a population health approach; to aid in this, it is critical to understand patients. Differences in population demographics and ethnic characteristics often lead to differences in risks, outcomes, and needs. By understanding these groups, the right care can be provided. Popular models to solve this issue are risk stratification and hierarchical diagnosis models. There are major limitations to these approaches as they tend to focus on high-use patients.[44] Also, they cannot deal with high-dimensional data.

An example of a clustering algorithm is k-means.[45] This algorithm clusters data into a predefined number of k clusters. There are then k centroids associated with each cluster. The algorithm's procedure is as follows:

- Select k points as initial centroids
- Repeat the following:
  - Form k clusters by assigning each point to its closest centroid
  - Re-compute the centroid of each cluster
    - If the centroid of each cluster does not change, do not repeat

The difficulty with implementing this algorithm is determining k, and outliers can unduly affect cluster assignment.

The following are example use cases:

- Calza et al. analyzed gene expression and clinical data to cluster 412 breast cancers and found that the algorithm could sort patients into five known subtypes of cancer.[46]

- Van der Laan et al. developed a patient segmentation algorithm to improve patient-centered care. They were able to segment patients into five categories: feeling vital, difficulties with psychosocial coping, physical and mobility complaints, difficulties experienced in multiple domains, and feeling extremely frail. They illustrated that there is an alignment with the patient categories and potential interventions.[47]
- Kaur et al. used a decision tree to predict diabetes with an accuracy rate of 99.87%.[48]

Advantages

Some of the biggest advantages of using the data mining technique are its robust validation methods and the way they are designed for generalizability. Building a model that fits the data you have and that can predict with high accuracy on the data you trained it with is not difficult with data mining tools. However, the more you fit your model to the data you have, the worse the prediction in real time usually is. Often one can build a model that fits the training data by making it more complex. However, that complexity makes it perform poorly when used for prediction in a real-world scenario. An easy example is that most decision tree algorithms default to producing a pruned tree, and that predicts better (usually) on unseen data than does an unpruned tree.

Modelers can use several different validation methods for supervised learning tasks. If you build a model that fits your training data, you still have no idea how it will perform on unseen data. It is ridiculously easy to build a highly accurate classifier that predicts accurately on the data used for training. One method for validation is splitting the data. You split the data into two sections (usually 66% and 33%). You train on the larger set and see how well it predicts on the smaller set. The gold standard method, however, is cross-validation. You split your data into partitions. Each partition is used multiple times for training and one time for testing. If you split into five groups, you will train and test five times. Each time you will use four partitions for training and one partition for testing. The model error is averaged across the iterations. Cross-validation gives a much better indication of the real-world error rate than does splitting.

Potential issues with data mining

There are several potential issues with using data mining tools in healthcare:

- Tools can be challenging to implement.
- Expertise is often missing.
- Some algorithms are so complicated it can be difficult to answer questions about the reason systems give the predictions they do.

- Data sets can have leaks where some of the features effectively give away the answer. Consider this scenario; you want to build a model to predict whether someone who has never had heart problems is likely to develop heart problems. You have a feature that lists whether they are on heart medication, and your model can use that to predict. That would bias your results because that feature is telling you whether someone already has heart problems.
- Healthcare data modeling and statistical issues often arise because data mining can be limited by the accessibility of data, because the raw inputs for data mining often exist in different settings and systems, such as administration, clinics, laboratories, and more. Hence, the data must be collected and integrated before data mining can be done and where other data problems may arise. These include missing, corrupted, inconsistent, or nonstandardized data, such as pieces of information recorded in different formats in different data sources. The lack of a standard clinical vocabulary is a serious hindrance to data mining. The quality of data mining results and applications depends on the quality of data.[49]

References

1. Hripcsak, G. et al. 2014. Health data use, stewardship, and governance: Ongoing gaps and challenges: A report from AMIA's 2012 health policy meeting. *Journal of the American Medical Informatics Association*, 21(2), 204–211.
2. Hersh, W. et al. 2011. Health-care hit or miss? *Nature*, 470(7334), 327–329.
3. Roski, J., Bo-Linn, G. W., Andrews, T. A. 2014. Creating value in health care through big data: Opportunities and policy implications. *Health Affairs (Project Hope)*, 33(7), 1115–1122.
4. Collins, S. A. et al. 2015. A practical approach to governance and optimization of structured data elements. In *MedInfo*, Washington D.C.: IOS Press, pp. 7–11. Available at: https://books.google.com/books?hl=en&lr=&id=OmZrCgAAQBAJ&oi=fnd&pg=PA7&dq=collins+medinfo+2015&ots=GAi1wfpNzF&sig=KgNxf-U5Y2JgHkvRlmKJ0i4P074#v=onepage&q=collins%20medinfo%202015&f=false
5. Williams, M. S., Ritchie, M. D., Payne, P. R. 2015. Interdisciplinary training to build an informatics workforce for precision medicine. *Applied and Translational Genomics*, 6, 28–30.
6. Data Governance Institute, Data Governance: The Basic Information. Available at: http://www.datagovernance.com/about/
7. Data quality techniques and best practices, *TechTarget*. Available at: https://searchdatamanagement.techtarget.com/definition/data-quality
8. Cohasset Associates. 2014. *Information Governance in Healthcare*. Chicago, IL: AHIMA.
9. Zozus, M. N., Bonner, J. 2017. Towards data value-level metadata for clinical studies. *Studies in Health Technology and Informatics*, 234, 418–423.
10. DeSalvo, K., Galvez, E. 2015. Connecting health and care for the nation: A shared nationwide interoperability roadmap-version 1.0. *Health IT Buzz*. Available at: https://www.healthit.gov/buzz-blog/electronic-health-and-medical-records/interoperability-electronic-health-and-medical-records/connecting-health-care-nation-shared-nationwide-interoperability-roadmap-version-10
11. KLAS Research. 2016. Interoperability 2016: From a Clinical View—Frustrating Reality or Hopeful Future. Orem, UT: KLAS Research.

12. Lenert, L., Sundwall, D., Lenert, M. E. 2012. Shifts in the architecture of the nationwide health information network. *Journal of the American Medical Informatics Association*, 19(4), 498–502.
13. Hersh, W. R. et al. 2015. Outcomes from health information exchange: Systematic review and future research needs. *JMIR Medical Informatics*, 3(4), e39.
14. HIMSS HIE Guide Work Group. *A HIMSS Guide to Participating in a Health Information Exchange*. Chicago, IL: HIMSS.
15. Health Level 7 International. 2012. HL7 EHR-S Vital Records Functional Profile, in *HL7 Standards Product Brief*. Available at: http://www.hl7.org
16. Mazouz, S., Malki, O. M. C., Nfaoui, E. H. 2015. Canonical document for medical data exchange. In: Yin, X. et al. (eds.), *Health Information Science*. HIS 2015. Lecture Notes in Computer Science (vol. 9085). Cham, Switzerland: Springer, pp. 37–44.
17. Nelson, E. C. et al. 2016. Patient focused registries can improve health, care, and science. *British Medical Journal*, 354, i3319.
18. Elliott, T. E., Holmes, J. H., Davidson, A. J., La Chance, P.-A., Nelson, A. F., Steiner, J. F. 2013. Data warehouse governance programs in healthcare settings: A literature review and a call to action. *Generating Evidence and Methods to Improve Patient Outcomes*, 1(1).
19. Black Book Market Research, December 20, 2016. 9 Healthcare Tech Trends in "The New Year of Uncertainty," Black Book Survey Results, *NEWSWIRE*, New York, NY.
20. Terrizzano, G., Schwarz, P. M., Roth, M., Colino, J. E. 2015. Data Wrangling: The Challenging Yourney from the Wild to the Lake, in *7th Biennial Conference on Innovative Data Systems Research (CIDR' 15)* January 4–7, 2015, Asilomar, California, USA.
21. Krause, D. D. 2015. Data lakes and data visualization: An innovative approach to address the challenges of access to health care in Mississippi. *Online Journal of Public Health Informatics*, 7(3).
22. Jannot, A.-S., Zapletal, E., Avillach, P., Mamzer, M.-F., Burgun, A., Degoulet, P. 2017. The Georges-Pompidou University hospital clinical data warehouse: A 8-years follow-up experience. *International Journal of Medical Informatics*, 102, 21–28.
23. Voss, E. A. et al. 2015. Feasibility and utility of applications of the common data model to multiple, disparate observational health databases. *Journal of the American Medical Informatics Association*, 22(3), 553–564.
24. HIMSS, HIMSS Health Story Project, *HIMSS*, May 3, 2016. Available at: http://www.himss.org/library/health-sto1y-project
25. Overhage, J. M., Ryan, P. B., Reich, C. G., Hartzema, A. G., Stang, P. E. 2012. Validation of a common data model for active safety surveillance research. *Journal of the American Medical Informatics Association*, 19(1), 54–60.
26. Reisinger, S. J. et al. 2012. Development and evaluation of a common data model enabling active drug safety surveillance using disparate healthcare databases. *Journal of the American Medical Informatics Association*, 652–662.
27. Gandomi, A., Haider, M. 2015. Beyond the hype: Big data concepts, methods, and analytics. *International Journal of Information Management*, 35(2), 137–144.
28. Jaroslav Pokorny. 2013. NoSQL databases: A step to database scalability in web environment. *International Journal on Semantic Web and Information Systems*, 9(1), 69–82.
29. White, T. 2015. *Hadoop: The Definitive Guide*, 4th ed. Beijing, China: O'Reilly Media.
30. Karau, H., Konwinski, A., Wendell, P., Zaharia, M. 2015. *Learning Spark: Lightning-Fast Big Data Analysis*. Boston, MA: O'Reilly Media.
31. Fayyad, U., Piatetsky-Shapiro, G., Smyth, P. 1996. From data mining to knowledge discovery in databases. *AI Magazine*, 17(3), 37.
32. Candelieri, A., Dolce, G., Riganello, F., Sannita, W. G. 2011. Data mining in neurology. In: *Knowledge-Oriented Applications in Data Mining*, K. Funatsu (ed.). London, UK: InTech.
33. Milovic, B. 2012. Usage of data mining in making business decision. *YU Info*, 153–157.

34. Yoo, I. et al. 2012. Data mining in healthcare and biomedicine: A survey of the literature. *Journal of Medical Systems*, 36(4), 2431–2448.
35. Hall, M. A., Holmes, G. 2003. Benchmarking attribute selection techniques for discrete class data mining. *IEEE Transactions on Knowledge and Data Engineering*, 15(6), 1437–1447.
36. Cheng, T. -H., Wei, C. -P., Tseng, V. S. 2006. Feature Selection for Medical Data Mining: Comparisons of Expert Judgment and Automatic Approaches, in *19th IEEE Symposium on Computer-Based Medical Systems (CBMS'06)*, 165–170.
37. Hastie, T., Tibshirani, R., Friedman, J. 2009. Overview of supervised learning. In: *The Elements of Statistical Learning*. Springer, New York, NY, pp. 9–41.
38. Safavian, S. R., Landgrebe, D. 1991. A survey of decision tree classifier methodology. *IEEE Transactions on Systems, Man, and Cybernetics*, 21(3), 660–674.
39. Raghupathi, W., Raghupathi, V. 2014. Big data analytics in healthcare: Promise and potential. *Health Information Science and Systems*, 2(1), 3.
40. Anbarasi, M., Anupriya, E., Iyengar, N. 2010. Enhanced prediction of heart disease with feature subset selection using genetic algorithm. *International Journal of Engineering, Science and Technology*, 2(10), 5370–5376.
41. Srinivas, K., Rani, B. K., Govrdhan, A. 2010. Applications of data mining techniques in healthcare and prediction of heart attacks. *International Journal of Computational Science and Engineering*, 2(02), 250–255.
42. Aggarwal, C. C., Reddy, C. K. 2013. *Data clustering: Algorithms and Applications*. Boca Raton, FL: CRC Press.
43. Using Population Segmentation to Provide Better Health Care for All: The "Bridges to Health" Model–LYNN–2007–The Milbank Quarterly–Wiley Online Library. Available at: http://onlinelibrary.wiley.com/doi/10.1 1 1 l/j.1468-0009.2007.00483.x/full
44. Vuik, S., Mayer, E., Darzi, A. 2016. Understanding population health needs: How data-driven population segmentation can support the planning of integrated care. *International Journal of Integrated Care*, 16(6).
45. Hartigan, J. A., Wong, M. A. 1979. Algorithm AS 136: A k-means clustering algorithm. *Journal of the Royal Statistical Society. Series C, Applied Statistics*, 28(1), 100–108.
46. Calza, S. et al. 2006. Intrinsic molecular signature of breast cancer in a population-based cohort of 412 patients. *Breast Cancer Research*, 8, R34.
47. Eissens van der Laan, M. R., van Offenbeek, M. A. G., Broekhuis, H., Slaets, J. P. J. 2014. A person-centred segmentation study in elderly care: Towards efficient demand-driven care. *Social Science and Medicine*, 113, 68–76.
48. Kaur, G., Chhabra, A. 2014. Improved J48 classification algorithm for the prediction of diabetes. *International Journal of Computer Applications*, 98(22).
49. Chopoorian, J. A., Witherell R., Khalil, O. E. M. Ahmed, M. 2001. Mind your business by mining your data. *SAM Advanced Management Journal*, 66(2), 45.

Chapter 5

Geospatial analysis of patients with healthcare utilization for type 2 diabetes mellitus (T2DM): A use case approach

Pradeep S. B. Podila

CONTENTS

Introduction

Diabetes mellitus (DM), the seventh leading cause of death in the United States, is a disease that affects millions of people each year[1] and claims more lives than both AIDS and breast cancer combined.[2] The prevalence of diabetes is on the rise due to aging, urbanization, and increasing prevalence of obesity and physical inactivity.

Diabetes is a very old disease and has been afflicting human beings for thousands of years. The first recorded writings documenting the disease came from an ancient Egyptian physician in 1552 BC who described the disease symptom of excessive urination.[3] The term *diabetes*, meaning "siphon" or "pass through" was coined in 250 BC. The term *mellitus* was first derived in the eleventh century from the Latin word for "honey." The first instances of testing for diabetes began with individuals referred to as "Water Tasters," who were responsible for diagnosing the disease by tasting urine to decide whether it was sweet or not.[4]

Diabetes affects the pancreas and results in limited usage of insulin or complete lack of insulin use in the body.[5] Insulin works as a hormonal agent in breaking down glucose so that it can be transitioned into energy for the body. There are two primary forms of diabetes that affect almost 30 million people across the nation, namely, type 1 DM (or T1DM) and type 2 DM (or T2DM). Children and young adults typically develop T1DM, which is tied to genetics; T2DM can

Table 5.1 Differences between Type 1 and Type 2 Diabetes Mellitus

	Type 1 Diabetes (T1DM)	Type 2 Diabetes (T2DM)
Age of Onset	Juvenile	Adult
Cause	No insulin	Insulin resistance, obesity
Prevalence	5%	95%
Symptoms	Severe	Less severe, obesity
Progression	Abrupt	Gradual
Consequences	Kidney, eyes, cardio	Kidney, eyes, cardio
Treatment	Insulin	Weight loss, diet control

be seen in a variety of populations, including children, but is more commonly diagnosed in older populations and characterized by excessive blood glucose levels. The differences between the two types of diabetes are better illustrated in Table 5.1.[6]

Burden of the disease

According to the American Diabetics Association, the prevalence of diabetes worldwide for all-age strata was estimated to increase from 2.8% in 2000 to 4.4% in 2030 (i.e., the total number of people with diabetes is projected to increase from 171 million in 2000 to 366 million in 2030, i.e., an increase of 114%).[7] T2DM is one of the most common noncommunicable diseases in the world today[8] and is becoming one of the most prevalent public health issues in the United States, with about 9.4% or 30.3 million adults diagnosed with the disease[9] and an additional 84.1 million people diagnosed with pre-diabetes, which usually translates into T2DM within 5 years. Research projects that by the year 2050, the prevalence of disease will increase by 54% to 54.9 million Americans, with associated costs rising to $622 billion annually.[10] The number of hospital discharges with diabetes as a principal diagnosis code increased from 454,000 in 1988 to 688,000 in 2009. An analysis of hospital discharge data in 2010 showed that patients with diabetes as a secondary diagnosis code or comorbidity accounted for about 62% or one-fourth of the encounters related to circulatory disorders. The number of U.S. adults aged 18 years or older diagnosed with diabetes almost quadrupled from 5.5 million in 1980 to 21.9 million in 2014.[11] In 1980, there were 5.6 million people with ages 18–79 years diagnosed with diabetes. By 2010, this number had increased to 20.9 million with the highest (25.2%) incidence noticed among people aged 65 years and older (i.e., Medicare patient population). The complications that arise from diabetes are a substantial source of morbidity and mortality.[12]

The disease has been spreading rapidly for the past decade and is following a similar trend as obesity, with a greater population of people with the disease located in the south and east. Tennessee ranked 42nd in the nation for median household income ($47,275) in 2015 and currently has the fifth highest diabetes rate in the nation, with 14.9% or 817,852 people diagnosed with the disease. Approximately 161,000 people in Tennessee do not realize that they have this disease and therefore are not taking care of their bodies properly. An additional 1.7 million people in Tennessee or 35.8% of the population have pre-diabetes and are at high risk for getting T2DM. With 38,000 people diagnosed with diabetes annually, Tennessee's diabetes rate is increasing faster than the diabetes rate in the United States, at 13% compared to 9%.[13] To further complicate the situation, about 16.7% of Tennessee residents live at or below the poverty level, and 17.6% rely on food stamps.[14] In 2012, Tennesseans spent a total of $4.9 billion on diabetes care alone in addition to the burden on financial status due to loss of productivity.

Memphis, which is the second most populous city in Tennessee, is located within Shelby County, which is the largest county in Tennessee by land area. Memphis has a higher prevalence of diabetes than the state average. Additionally, Memphis' diabetes patients have the highest A1C levels out of all major Tennessee cities, with 20.8% of T2DM patients having a higher glucose or blood sugar (i.e., A1C) level.[15] In 2004, 9.2% of the Shelby County residents were living with diabetes, and this number had risen to 12.2% by 2013, which is actually one of the lowest in the state.[16] However, this glimmer of hope diminishes when we observe the diabetes-related mortality rate in Shelby County (Figure 5.1) of 28.9% compared to the national mortality rate of 23.1%,[17] which begs the necessity of analyzing the T2DM hospitalization rates to better understand this patient population in order to design targeted interventions.

Research question

Although geographical information systems (GISs) have been widely used in various industries, they have not been used by healthcare entities due to the challenges related to patient data privacy/security and the complexity of handling a multitude of data sources. This could change quickly due to the growing importance of population health and precision medicine. The elements of epidemiological planning models,[18] such as overall population, population at risk, and socioeconomic characteristics, play a key role in the road to population health, which can be further enhanced by including the spatial component (i.e., location of the patient in relation to the healthcare entity). Although the disparities related to racial and socioeconomic factors in the context of diabetes have been widely published, it is very important to understand the burden at a local or spatial level when designing interventions targeted at high-risk and vulnerable patient populations.

The purpose of this example is twofold: (1) show the burden of diabetes in the mid-South region, which is often referred to as the "capital for many chronic diseases"

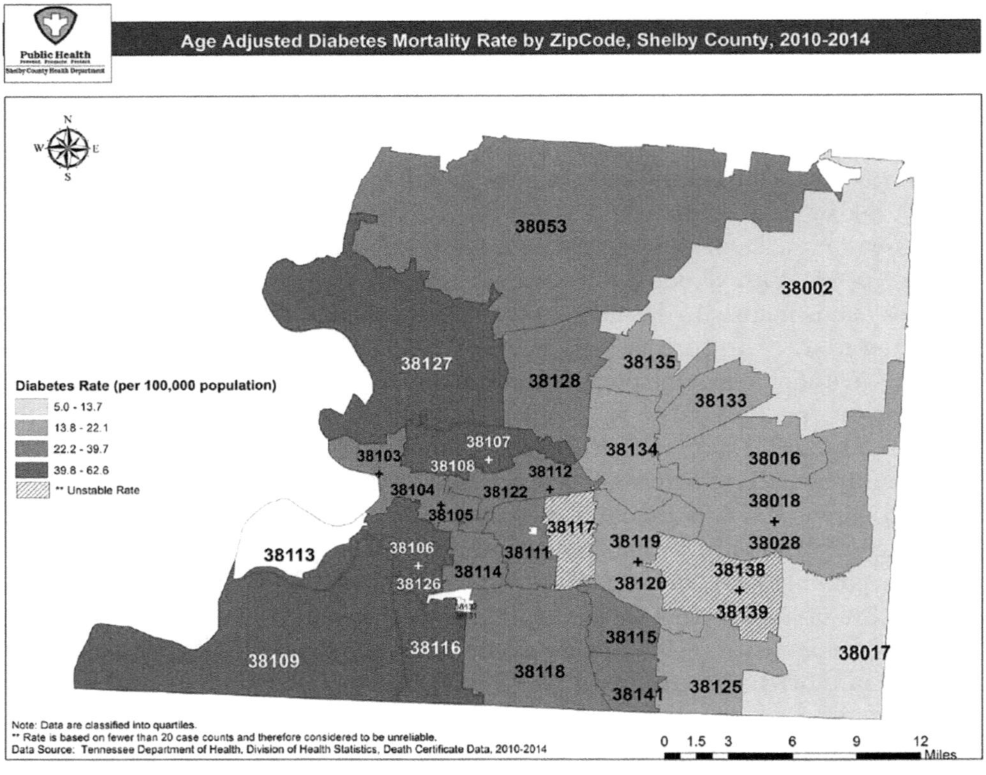

Figure 5.1 Diabetes mortality rates in Shelby County, Tennessee, 2010–2014.

and (2) demonstrate how the GIS analysis of the same data provides added value by educating the key stakeholders such as community leaders, local hospitals, and the local county health department about the spatial disparities related to T2DM.

Materials and methods

Study site

Methodist Le Bonheur Healthcare (MLH) is a large, not-for-profit, integrated healthcare delivery system based in Memphis, Tennessee, generating in excess of $1.2 billion in operating revenues. Founded in 1918 by the United Methodist Church to help meet the growing needs for quality healthcare in the mid-South, MLH is a six-hospital system (Figure 5.2), with a free-standing nationally renowned children's hospital and an academic medical center affiliated with the University of Tennessee Health Science Center (UTHSC) and controlling 47% of the local market share. We have only included the encounters of those aged 18 years and older from the adult hospitals in this analysis.

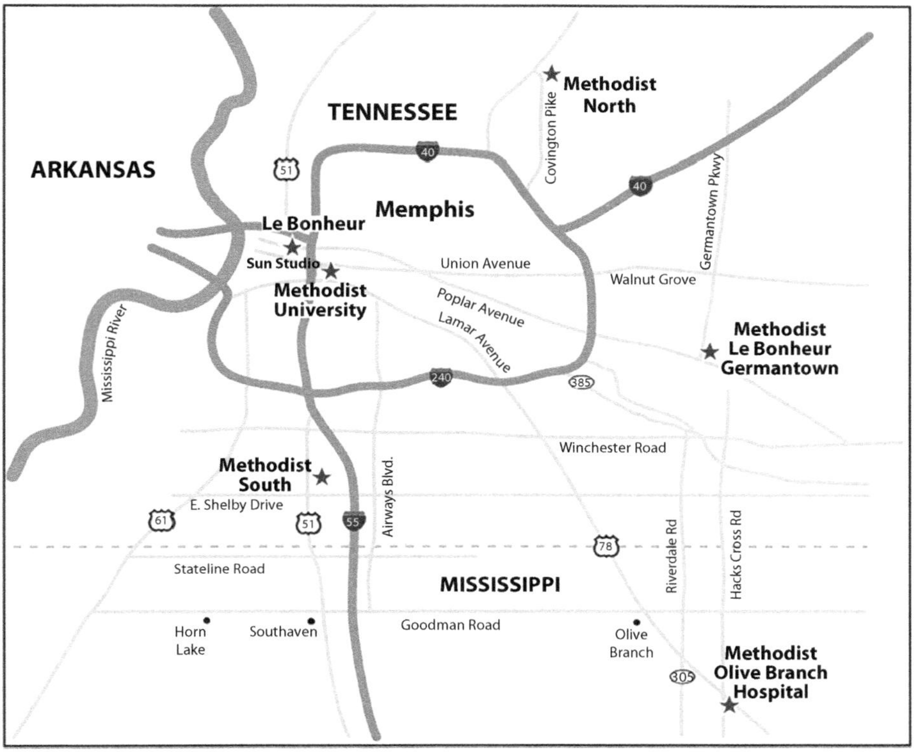

Figure 5.2 MLH facilities.

Study design and approval

A retrospective longitudinal study was performed on the medical records of the patients who have been discharged from an inpatient (hospitalization) status with a primary T2DM diagnosis between January 1, 2007, and December 31, 2013, from MLH. The 7-year timeline (2007–2013) followed the *International Classification of Diseases, Ninth Revision, Clinical Modification* (*ICD-9-CM*) standards set forth for classifying the discharges for various disease conditions. The diagnosis codes of T2DM (classified by *ICD-9-CM* as 250.XX) used in the current study are provided in Table 5.2.

The data set used in this study (14-02937-XM) was approved by the Institutional Review Board (IRB) at the University of Tennessee Health Science Center (UTHSC), Methodist Healthcare Memphis Hospitals (MHMH), and the University of Memphis (UofM) as a part of the all-cause readmissions research project.

Data elements

Demographics, primary and secondary diagnosis codes, number of acute visits (emergency department [ED], and outpatient [OP]), short hospitalizations (<24 hours,

Table 5.2 ICD-9-CM Type 2 Diabetes Mellitus (T2DM) diagnosis codes

Diagnosis code	Diagnosis description
250.00	DM without mention of complication, type 2 or unspecified type, not stated as uncontrolled
250.02	DM without mention of complication, type 2 or unspecified type, uncontrolled
250.10	DM with ketoacidosis, type 2 or unspecified type, not stated as uncontrolled
250.12	DM with ketoacidosis, type 2 or unspecified type, uncontrolled
250.20	DM with hyperosmolarity, type 2 or unspecified type, not stated as uncontrolled
250.22	DM with hyperosmolarity, type 2 or unspecified type, uncontrolled
250.30	DM with other coma, type 2 or unspecified type, not stated as uncontrolled
250.32	DM with other coma, type 2 or unspecified type, uncontrolled
250.40	DM with renal manifestations, type 2 or unspecified type, not stated as uncontrolled
250.42	DM with renal manifestations, type 2 or unspecified type, uncontrolled
250.50	DM with ophthalmic manifestations, type 2 or unspecified type, not stated as uncontrolled
250.52	DM with ophthalmic manifestations, type 2 or unspecified type, uncontrolled
250.60	DM with neurological manifestations, type 2 or unspecified type, not stated as uncontrolled
250.62	DM with neurological manifestations, type 2 or unspecified type, uncontrolled
250.70	DM with peripheral circulatory disorders, type 2 or unspecified type, not stated as uncontrolled
250.72	DM with peripheral circulatory disorders, type 2 or unspecified type, uncontrolled

(*Continued*)

Table 5.2 (*Continued*) ICD-9-CM Type 2 Diabetes Mellitus (T2DM) diagnosis codes

250.80	DM with other specified manifestations, type 2 or unspecified type, not stated as uncontrolled
250.82	DM with other specified manifestations, type 2 or unspecified type, uncontrolled
250.90	DM with unspecified complication, type 2 or unspecified type, not stated as uncontrolled
250.92	DM with unspecified complication, type 2 or unspecified type, uncontrolled

i.e., OBS), hospitalizations (inpatient [IP]), 30-day hospital readmissions, and street address/city/zip code were extracted and collected for all patients. The median household income at zip code level from the American Community Survey (ACS) (2006–2010) retrieved from the Michigan Population Studies Center was used as a proxy to assess patients' income level.

The original data set had 6,435 inpatient hospitalizations with a principal or primary diagnosis of T2DM from 4,643 unique patients (i.e., 1.4 encounters per patient). These encounters are from residents of all counties (including Shelby County) who had encounters at MLH. To identify the unique characteristics (i.e., factors associated with the utilization of these T2DM patients), we have only considered their very first encounter for T2DM within the entire data set as the baseline or index encounter.

Descriptive and spatial statistics

The descriptive statistics were computed using SAS version 9.3 (Cary, North Carolina), and the spatial clusters were identified using Getis-Ord Gi* statistic within the ESRI ArcMap 10.5.1 (Redlands, California).

Subject selection by geospatial analysis

The spatial unit of analysis used to analyze the descriptive and utilization characteristics of T2DM patients is the geocoded residential addresses (individual-level measure) of all unique cases (i.e., baseline or index encounter). The geocoding was performed on the de-identified baseline or index spatial data elements of the 4,643 patients. The comma delimited (.csv) file with the minimum required spatial data elements—de-identified identifier, street address, city, state, and five-digit zip code—was submitted at the U.S. Census Bureau Address Batch geocoder module to generate the geolocation of the records (i.e., corresponding latitude, longitude, match [Match or No Match], type of match [Exact or Non Exact], state, and county codes).

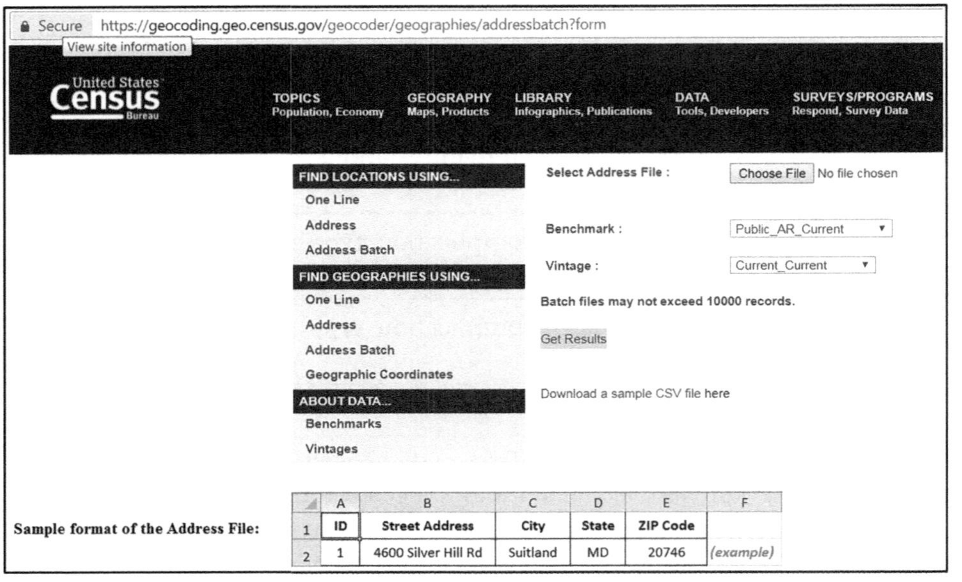

Figure 5.3 Geocoding settings and the ample format inout address file.

Please note that the input data file to the Address Batch geocoder only needs the data (i.e., no header information is required) but should strictly follow the sequence of the fields for generating accurate results. The geocoding settings and the sample format of the address file are provided in Figure 5.3.

The de-identified geospatial data was attached back to the original data set based on the ID and to identify the Shelby County (Code: 47) residents. Following this, the Hotspot Analysis tool (Getis-Ord Gi*) within ArcGIS 10.5.1 along with the Kriging, an advanced geospatial procedure to generate the estimated surface area (~5,000 meters), were used to identify the clusters or regions of patients with T2DM encounters. The Getis-Ord Gi* was used to compute the statistically significant positive z-scores (the larger the z-score) to identify the more intense clustering of high values (i.e., hot spots). As displayed in Figure 5.4, the analysis generated four clusters, but only two of them circled in black stood out within the 99% confidence interval, i.e., of the 4,643 patients in the original data set, 73.3% or 3,405 patients with encounters at MLH were Shelby County residents who fell within the high-intense spatial clusters for T2DM (Cluster 1 = 2,803 patients, and Cluster 2 = 602 patients).

Results

The 4,643 unique patients in the original data set had 6,435 inpatient hospitalizations with a principal or a primary diagnosis of T2DM (i.e., 1.4 encounters per patient). The same patients had 54,197 encounters (including inpatient, emergency, observation,

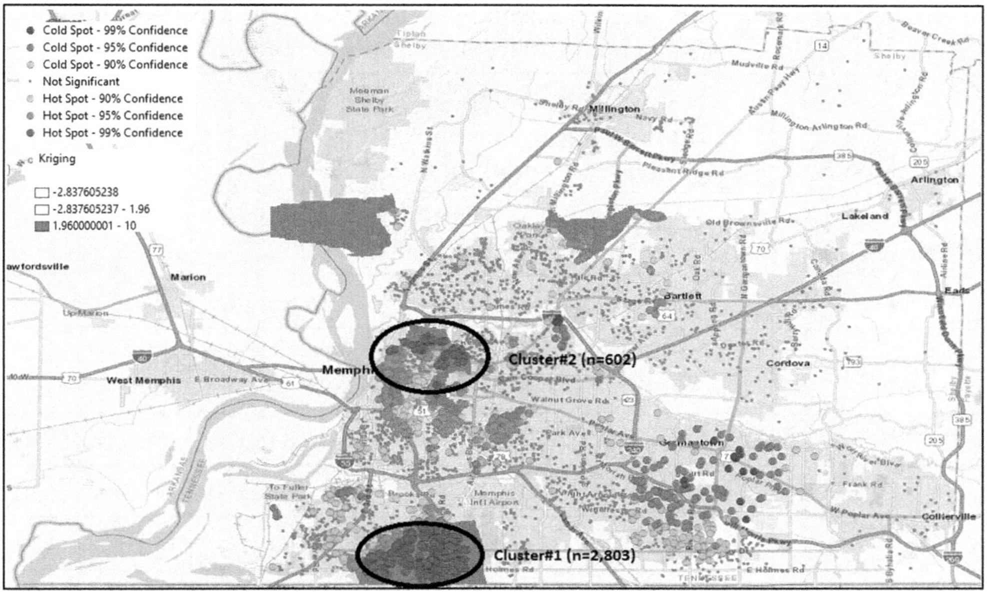

Figure 5.4 Spatial clusters of T2DM patients.

and outpatient) during the 7-year period, i.e., 11.7 encounters per patient, which is almost 10 times that of their diabetes-related encounters. This clearly highlights the importance and significance of the study to better understand the characteristics of this patient population.

In Table 5.3, we notice that the mean age of the patients across the different comparison groups was in the range of 56 years. But, when the age strata are taken into consideration, there was a slight increase (~2%) in the number of individuals within the age group of 45–64 years in Cluster 2 compared to those within the other clusters. Cluster 2 had a higher representation of females (~55%) compared to Cluster 1 (~51%), and African Americans (~94%) compared to Cluster 1 (~78%). Interestingly, among the patients on Medicare, we have noticed a difference of about 2.6% between the clusters (Cluster 1 = 44.3% versus Cluster 2 = 41.7%); and an opposite trend on those on Charity Care (Cluster 1 = 17.1% versus Cluster 2 = 20.1%). When compared to Cluster 1, Cluster 2 was predominantly represented by the patients with a median household income less than $40,000 measured at the zip code level.

In Table 5.4, we notice that when compared to the original data set, the overall healthcare utilization of the T2DM patients within both the clusters was higher in all aspects related to healthcare utilization, i.e., emergency visits, observation stays, inpatient hospitalizations, and 30-day readmissions. Interestingly, Table 5.5 showed that the diabetes-related utilization, i.e., average encounters per patient, was similar to that of those in the original data set.

Table 5.3 Demographic and socioeconomic characteristics of patients with a principal or primary diagnosis of T2DM

Variable	Original data set	Clusters 1 and 2 combined	Cluster 1	Cluster 2
Total Sample (n)	4,643	3,405	2,803 (82.3%)	602 (17.7%)
Age (years)	57.4±16.1	56.6±16.3	56.7±16.3	56.4±16.0
Age Group (years)				
18–44	1,001 (21.6)	785 (23.1)	650 (23.2)	135 (22.4)
45–64	2,069 (44.6)	1,514 (44.5)	1,237 (44.1)	277 (46.0)
65+	1,573 (33.9)	1,106 (32.5)	916 (32.7)	190 (31.6)
Gender				
Female	2,375 (51.2)	1,780 (52.3)	1,448 (51.7)	332 (55.1)
Male	2,265 (48.8)	1,623 (47.7)	1,353 (48.3)	270 (44.9)
Race				
African American	3.496 (75.3)	2,745 (80.6)	2,180 (77.8)	565 (93.9)
Caucasian	1,040 (22.4)	580 (17.0)	553 (19.7)	27 (4.5)
Insurance Type				
Medicare	2,233 (48.1)	1,494 (43.9)	1,243 (44.3)	251 (41.7)
Medicaid/ Tenncare	516 (11.1)	387 (11.4)	318 (11.3)	69 (11.5)
Charity	728 (15.7)	600 (17.6)	479 (17.1)	121 (20.1)
Commercial	1,134 (24.4)	924 (27.1)	748 (26.7)	161 (26.7)
Median Household Income ($)*	39,195± 17,084	38,205± 17,514	39,399± 18,717	32,646± 8,148
<20,000	99 (2.1)	74 (2.2)	34 (1.2)	40 (6.6)

(*Continued*)

Table 5.3 (*Continued*) Demographic and socioeconomic characteristics of patients with a principal or primary diagnosis of T2DM

20,000–40,000	3,274 (70.5)	2,601 (76.4)	2,047 (73.0)	554 (92.0)
40,000–60,000	668 (14.4)	310 (9.1)	305 (10.9)	5 (0.8)
≥60,000	562 (12.1)	420 (12.3)	417 (14.9)	3 (0.5)

Note: Categorical variables are presented as No. (%) and continuous measures as mean ± standard deviation.
*Median Household Income at zip code level was obtained from American Community Survey (ACS).

Table 5.4 Overall healthcare utilization of the patients with a principal or primary diagnosis of T2DM

Visit type	Original data set (n=4,643 patients)	Clusters 1 and 2 combined (n=3,405 patients)	Cluster 1 (n=2,803 patients)	Cluster 2 (n=602 patients)
Emergency Department	20,945 (4.5)	16,240 (6.1)	13,218 (6.0)	3,022 (6.4)
Observation (<24 hours)	2,204 (0.5)	1,667 (1.8)	1,352 (1.8)	315 (1.8)
Inpatient (hospitalization)	21,483 (4.6)	16,226 (4.8)	13,269 (4.7)	2,957 (4.9)
Outpatient	9,565 (2.1)	6,995 (3.8)	5,846 (3.8)	1,149 (3.6)
Total Encounters	54,197 (11.7)	41,128 (12.1)	33,685 (12.0)	7,443 (12.4)
30-day Inpatient Readmissions*	5,452 (3.1)	4,123 (1.9)	3,363 (3.2)	760 (3.2)

*Total No. of encounters (Average encounters per patient) or Total No. of readmissions (Average readmissions per patient).

Discussion

The U.S. healthcare system currently spends almost 9% of its total spending on the direct treatment of diabetes. To further complicate the matters, according to the Centers for Disease Control and Prevention (CDC) approximately 7.2 million people in the United States do not even realize that they have diabetes; from the

Table 5.5 Diabetes-related healthcare utilization of the patients

Visit type	Original data set ($n = 4,643$ patients)	Clusters 1 and 2 combined ($n = 3,405$ patients)	Cluster 1 ($n = 2,803$ patients)	Cluster 2 ($n = 602$ patients)
Emergency Department	1,645 (1.8)	1,276 (1.7)	1,022 (1.7)	254 (1.7)
Observation (<24 hours)	277 (1.2)	216 (1.2)	175 (1.2)	41 (1.2)
Inpatient (hospitalization)	6,435 (1.4)	4,756 (1.4)	3,851 (1.4)	905 (1.5)
Outpatient	199 (1.2)	136 (1.2)	117 (1.2)	19 (1.1)
Total Encounters	8,556 (1.8)	6,384 (1.9)	5,165 (1.8)	1,219 (2.0)
30-day Inpatient Readmissions*	1,112 (1.5)	819 (1.5)	651 (1.5)	168 (1.5)

*Total No. of encounters (Average encounters per patient) or Total No. of readmissions (Average readmissions per patient).

current use case, we have noticed that patients with T2DM have a 10-fold higher healthcare utilization across the board, i.e., emergency visits, observation stays, inpatient hospitalizations/readmissions, and outpatient visits for both diabetes- and non-diabetes-related encounters. The descriptive data exploration coupled with GIS hot spot analysis has revealed the stark gender, racial, insurance, and income disparities among the patients within the high-concentration clusters. This information can be valuable for key stakeholders in fostering alliances and collaborations at a community level toward developing place-based interventions to curtail unnecessary healthcare utilization, thereby reducing the overall burden of the disease.

As the United States spends the greatest gross domestic product (GDP) (17.9%)[19] on healthcare in the world, diabetes management has been identified by both the U.S. Department of Health and Human Services (DHHS) and the CDC as a very important mission toward minimizing the long-term consequences associated with diabetes, such as kidney disease, nerve damage, retinal disease, heart disease, and stroke. Patients with diabetes were also the greatest contributors to the high overall unplanned 30-day hospital readmission rates, which is a performance measure used by the CMS to adjust reimbursements for overall Medicare discharges. This use case demonstrated the utility of GIS to better understand the characteristics of patients at a spatial level, i.e., within the highly concentrated clusters of healthcare utilization within a hospital's market service area.

References

1. Centers for Disease Control and Prevention (CDC). 2017. *National Diabetes Statistics Report, 2017. Estimates of Diabetes and Its Burden in the United States.*
2. Edelman, D. April, 2017. Why Do Cancer and AIDS Get More Support Than Diabetes? Available at: https://www.diabetesdaily.com/blog/2013/03/why-do-canceraids-get-more-support-than-diabetes/
3. Swidorski, D. March 14, 2014. Diabetes History. Available at: https://www.defeatdiabetes.org/diabetes-history/
4. Diabetes Activist. January 6, 2017. History of Diabetes. Available at: http://www.diabetesactivist.com/a-little-history/
5. National Institute of Diabetes and Digestive and Kidney Diseases. November, 2016. What Is Diabetes? Available at: https://www.niddk.nih.gov/health-information/diabetes/overview/what-is-diabetes
6. From a conversation with Tyra, A. 2017. Problem Statement: Diabetes. University of Memphis, School of Public Health, Memphis, TN. Managerial Epidemiology student.
7. Wild, S., Roglic, G., Green, A., Sicree, R., King, H. 2004. Global prevalence of diabetes: Estimates for the year 2000 and projections for 2030. *Diabetes Care*. 2004 May, 27(5), 1047–1053.
8. Amos, A. F., McCarty, D. J., Zimmet, P. 1997. The Rising Global Burden of Diabetes and Its Complications: Estimates and Projections to the Year 2010. *Diabetic Medicine*, 14, S1–85.
9. Centers for Disease Control and Prevention. May, 2017. Health, United States, 2016. Available at: https://www.cdc.gov/nchs/data/hus/hus16.pdf#019
10. Rowley, W. R., Bezold, C., Arikan, Y., Byrne, E., Krohe, S. 2017. Diabetes 2030: Insights from Yesterday, Today, and Future Trends. *Population Health Management*. February 1, 2017, 20(1), 6–12.
11. Rana, J. S. 2016. Is Diabetes Really a CHD Risk Equivalent? Available at: http://www.acc.org/latest-in-cardiology/articles/2016/04/12/13/40/is-diabetes-really-a-chd-risk-equivalent
12. Geraghty, E. M., Balsbaugh, T., Nuovo, J., Tandon, S. 2010. Using Geographical Information Systems (GIS) to assess outcome disparities in patients with type 2 diabetes and hyperlipidemia. *Journal of the American Board of Family Medicine*, 23(1), 88–96.
13. American Diabetes Association (ADA). 2016. The Burden of Diabetes in Tennessee. Available at: http://main.diabetes.org/dorg/PDFs/Advocacy/burden-of-diabetes/tennessee.pdf
14. Frohlich, T. C., Sauter, M. B., Stebbins, S. 2016. America's Richest (and Poorest) States. Available at: http://247wallst.com/special-report/2016/09/15/americas-richest-and-poorest-states-4/3/
15. IMS Health. 2016. Type 2 Diabetes Report 2016: Tennessee. Available at: http://www.hc21.org/pdfs/Tenn_HC21_MemphisBGH_2015D2.pdf
16. Charlier, T. 2017, March 11. Programs help blunt Memphis' diabetes epidemic. Commercial Appeal. Available at: http://www.commercialappeal.com/story/news/health/2017/03/11/programs-help-blunt-memphis-diabetes-epidemic/98091046/
17. Shelby County Health Department (SCHD). 2015. Shelby County, TN Community Health Assessment. Available at: https://www.shelbycountytn.gov/DocumentCenter/View/22144
18. White, K. R., Griffith, J. R. 2010. *The Well-Managed Healthcare Organization*, 7th ed. Chicago, IL: Health Administration Press.
19. Centers for Medicare and Medicaid Services. 2017. National Health Expenditures 2016 Highlights. Available at: https://www.cms.gov/Research-Statistics-Data-and-Systems/Statistics-Trends-and-Reports/NationalHealthExpendData/downloads/highlights.pdf

Chapter 6

Futuring: A brief overview of methods and tools

Ross M. Mullner

CONTENTS

According to the popular science fiction writer and futurist Isaac Asimov, "Predicting the future is a hopeless, thankless task, with ridicule to begin with and, all too often, scorn to end with."[1]

Despite the daunting task of forecasting and predicting the future, major future changes must be anticipated and planned for by individuals, organizations, and governments.

Without the appropriate planning, individuals will have a very difficult time adjusting to and navigating within the future changes, organizations that do not evolve and accept the future changes will fail and close, and governments that do not develop new policies and laws addressing future changes will not be effective, efficient, equitable, or economic.

The future is so very difficult to forecast and predict because it is dynamically complex. It includes a vast array of potential changes, many of which interact and cause other changes. Major future changes can occur in the physical environment (e.g., global warming and rising sea levels), demographics (decline in the number of children and the growth of the elderly), societies (increasing modernity and the decline in formal religions), cultures (decline in the number of native languages and the Westernization of the Third World), economics (worldwide depressions and recessions), politics (increasing polarization and the rise of conservatism), and technologies (the development of new drugs, and the increasing use of computers and robotics in medicine).[2–4]

Future changes may occur slowly or quickly, and they may be constant or dramatic in nature. Further, although it is difficult to forecast and predict changes in the near future (less than 5 years), it is even harder to accurately forecast and predict changes in the long-term future (5 years or more).

One example of a major long-term future change that is constant and occurring slowly is the aging of the world's population. According to the United Nations, virtually every country in the world is experiencing growth in the number and proportion of older persons in their population. This demographic future change will be one of the most significant social transformations of the twenty-first century. The aging of the population is already having major implications for society, including the demand for goods and services, especially healthcare services, housing, transportation, labor and financial markets, as well as family structure and intergenerational ties.[5]

Another major long-term future change that is occurring is the quick technological advances taking place in healthcare. Such advances include the increasing use of wearable tracking devices to monitor physical activity, caloric consumption, and sleep activities by the general public; a much greater emphasis on patient-centered care by hospitals and other healthcare facilities; a greater emphasis on patient data security; and ever-increasing data demands by patients, insurance companies, and the federal and state governments.[6,7]

To better understand possible future changes and emerging trends, a new field of study has evolved known as futuring. Although definitions vary, futuring can be very broadly defined as the process of using a systematic process for thinking about and picturing possible outcomes and planning for the future. Looking at trends, patterns, and historical information, futurists attempt to forecast and predict possible and probable futures.[8,9]

The largest and oldest individual membership organization representing futurists is the World Future Society. Founded in 1966, and headquartered in Chicago, Illinois, the not-for-profit World Future Society currently has approximately 40,000 members worldwide. Past members have included such notables as Buckminster Fuller, Herman Kahn, Gene Roddenberry, and Margaret Mead. The society holds an annual national meeting, and it produces online newsletters and publications for its members.

Another influential futurist organization is the Institute for the Future. Founded in 1968 as a spin-off from the RAND Corporation, and headquartered in Palo Alto, California, the not-for-profit Institute for the Future works with companies, governments, and individuals to help them plan for the long-term future. The institute makes long-term forecasts and develops maps for three broad areas: global trends, people and technology, and health and healthcare. It divides its healthcare area into four parts: health futures, healthcare, health games, and aging. A few examples of the institute's current health and healthcare forecasts and maps, all of which are available online, include "Health Aware World Map," "Booting Up Mobile Health," "A New Era of Diagnostics," "The Futuring of Pharmaceuticals," and "Caregiving 2031."

Futurists use a number of methods and tools to forecast and predict future changes. Forecasts differ from predictions. Specifically, forecasts are a set of possible futures that often include probability estimates of events occurring at some generalized time point. For example, futurists might attempt to forecast what the nation's healthcare system will be like 25 years in the future. In contrast, predictions are estimates of specific events or numbers at a particular time in the future. Futurists might predict what percentage of the U.S. gross domestic product (GDP) will be spent on healthcare in the year 2030. It should be noted that forecasts may consist of a set of predictions with associated probabilities.

The four most common methods and tools used by futurists to forecast and predict future change include statistical regression models, Delphi survey technique, environmental scanning—SWOT analysis, and scenario analysis. Each method and tool along with its strengths and weaknesses is discussed in the following sections.

Statistical regression models

Statistical regression models are the most basic and commonly used method to predict or estimate a number in the future. Regression models are frequently used in business, economics, sociology, medicine, and public health, especially epidemiology. These models are used to calculate an estimate of a future change, identify the influence and importance of factors or variables associated with the change being predicted, and calculate the predicted degree of risk of an adverse event.[10]

Although there are many types of statistical regression models (i.e., linear, logistic, polynomial, stepwise, ridge, lasso, and elastic net regression), the most common type is linear regression, and the most common type of linear regression is ordinary least squares regression.[11]

Regression models can be simple or complex. A simple regression model has one independent variable to predict a dependent variable. In contrast, a multiple regression model has many independent variables to explain or predict a dependent variable.[12]

Statistical regression models can be used as time series tools predicting a future number based on past numbers using time as a variable. For example, a hospital administrator may want to use a simple regression model to predict a hospital's future inpatient admissions. Monthly data from the past several years could be gathered and plotted on a graph. These data then could be entered into an Excel or other online program, and a regression line could be calculated and fitted to the data. This would enable the administrator to estimate or predict the anticipated number of inpatients the hospital will treat next month or for several months or even years into the future.

Very complex multiple logistic regression models are often used in medicine and public health to calculate the risk of an adverse or negative event. In this type of model, the dependent variable is generally a dichotomous outcome—the patient survived or died, a medical error occurred or did not occur, and the patient or resident fell or did not fall.[13]

For example, a healthcare administrator might want to predict the risk of a patient or resident suffering a fall at his or her facility. Fatal falls, especially among the elderly, are an important medical and public health problem. And many older individuals in hospitals and nursing homes fall. To identify and predict the risk of falling, a multiple logistic regression model could be constructed. The model would include many independent variables as possible explanatory factors, such as how and when the patient or resident was admitted; their age, gender, and race; the number and types of medical conditions they have; the number and types of medication they receive; and what floor or unit provided care to them. The dependent variable would be whether they fell during their stay or not. The model would predict the risk of falling for each individual, and a comparison could be made to see who actually did fall. If the model predicts well, a score could be given to new patients entering the facility, and individuals with a high likelihood of falling in the future could be more closely monitored and provided more appropriate care.[14]

Strengths and weaknesses

Regression models can be used in many situations, and they are very powerful tools to predict the future. They have the advantage of being widely used and well known.

Researchers have many resources available to them to use this statistical tool. There are numerous textbooks on the subject and many educational resources online and at local colleges and universities.

However, regression models also have a number of problems. Because they are so widely available, many researchers tend to ignore the underlying assumptions of the models, which vary by the type of regression used. Researchers often do not specify the model well. They frequently use the wrong independent variables to make their predictions, leading to weak or biased estimates and bad predictions. And researchers often falsely conclude that a statistical correlation is causation.

Delphi survey technique

Futurists often use the Delphi survey technique to forecast the future. The basic underlying assumption of this technique is that experts in a field of study know the most about the field, and they will make the best and most accurate forecasts within the field. Named after the Oracle of Delphi of Greek mythology, the Delphi survey technique was developed by the RAND Corporation in the 1950s. The technique was initially used to forecast various questions concerning the impact of technology on warfare. Over the years, the Delphi survey technique has been widely used by businesses, associations, research organizations, governments, and healthcare systems.[15] The Delphi technique consists of a series of systematic interactive steps to derive a consensus from a panel of independent experts. To begin the process, a facilitator develops an initial questionnaire that broadly outlines the question or questions of interest. A panel of independent experts is then selected, often consisting of 15–20 individuals. Each expert is given the questionnaire and asked to complete the survey anonymously. The facilitator then gathers, compiles, and summarizes the responses. The summary is then given to each panel expert, and they are again asked to respond. This process (or rounds) continues three or more times, reducing the range of responses until an expert consensus of opinion is derived.[16]

In the past, panels of experts were brought to a research facility or central location for several days or weeks, where they were given the surveys. Today, the panels of experts are often sent the surveys by e-mail and asked to respond by certain dates.

The Delphi survey technique has been widely used in healthcare to standardize health outcome measures, identify key components of healthcare problems, and identify, refine, and rate success factors and various performance measures. The Delphi technique has also been used to forecast likely new medical technology and future changes in the U.S. healthcare delivery system.[17]

Strengths and weaknesses

If the Delphi survey technique is used appropriately, it can be a versatile, fast, and cost-effective forecasting tool. Using e-mail, the technique has the advantage of bringing together a very geographically dispersed panel of independent experts. The technique allows their responses to be confidential and avoids direct confrontation between experts.

However, the technique also has a number of problems. There are no guidelines for determining consensus. It is also not clear how many independent experts should be chosen for a panel. Depending on the size and complexity of the survey, it may require a major time commitment, which the experts may not be willing to spend. Some experts may also take a long time to respond or even drop out of the study. Last, a number of researchers have seriously questioned the overall reliability of the Delphi survey technique.

Environmental scanning: SWOT analysis

Many businesses, not-for-profit organizations, government units, universities, hospitals, health systems, and healthcare associations conduct environmental scans. For example, many large health systems conduct periodic environmental scans, while the American Hospital Association conducts a yearly environmental scan that it publishes and widely distributes to its member hospitals and the general public.[18]

Environment scans are often used by the various organizations to conduct SWOT analyses. SWOT is an acronym that stands for strengths, weaknesses, opportunities, and threats. Organizations conduct SWOT analyses to identify what they do well, where they can improve, how they fit in the competitive landscape, and how they can better position themselves in the near and distant future. They also frequently use SWOT analyses to evaluate their programs, products, and services they provide.[19]

Environmental scans are used in the strategic planning process to identify broad issues and trends that will have important implications for the organization's future. Organizations generally conduct both internal and external environmental scans. The degree to which the internal environmental scan matches the external environmental scan identifies the degree of strategic fit of an organization.

Organizations scan their internal environment by conducting a self-assessment to identify such issues as overall worker satisfaction, employee turnover rates, sources of income, the age of buildings and equipment, and customer and patient satisfaction.

They scan the external environment, which for healthcare organizations often includes consumer and patient characteristics (e.g., consumer and patient expectations, overall healthcare spending, and medical conditions); economy and finance issues (e.g., changes in Medicare and Medicaid policies, and problems in paying healthcare bills); information technology and e-health (e.g., data breaches and information security); insurance and coverage changes (e.g., growth of insurance exchanges and subsidies and tax credits); workforce and physician issues (e.g., future supply and demand for nurses and physicians); government and politics (e.g., federal policy changes and state healthcare policy changes); provider organizations (e.g., health systems and Accountable Care Organizations); and quality and patient safety issues (e.g., improvements in coordination of care activities, medical errors, and changes in hospital-acquired conditions).

The environmental scans are then used to conduct a SWOT analysis. The four factors of SWOT are combined into a matrix, which helps organizations make strategic decisions about their future. SWOT analysis is also frequently used to evaluate units of organizations and various programs. For example, SWOT recently was used to evaluate e-health advances to support people with multiple medical conditions and complex healthcare needs at sites in Canada, Scotland, and the United States. The analysis helped the authors develop a number of recommendations that will help each of the countries implement more effective programs in the future.[20]

Strengths and weaknesses

The environmental scanning tool has a number of strengths. It can help organizations and programs identify emerging opportunities that can be capitalized on, ensure the appropriate strategy to better fit emerging conditions, and help avoid costly mistakes. However, the tool has several weaknesses: it is difficult to judge the amount of resources necessary to conduct the scans, and interpretation of the fast-changing environment is a very inexact science at best.

SWOT analysis also has strengths and weaknesses. Its main strengths are its simplicity and cost effectiveness. Because the method does not require a high degree of technical skill or training, almost any staff member can be picked to conduct the analysis. However, SWOT analysis does have a number of weaknesses, including that it has no mechanism to rank the significance or weight of the various factors (all of the factors are considered of equal importance); it is a simple, one-dimensional model with each factor allocated to only one category; and the data used for the analysis may be outdated (many statistics are years old).

Scenario analysis

Futurists often make forecasts of the distant future using scenario analysis. Scenarios are stories describing possible ways the future may unfold. The scenarios bound the uncertainty of the future into a limited number of likely paths. Scenario analysis is widely used to manage risk and develop strategic plans for the future. Both the private and public sectors use scenario analysis. Corporations use it to manage large capital investments and change and modify their corporate strategies, while public sector agencies tend to use it to plan for population growth and regional development. In the developing world, nations use scenario analysis to identify opportunities, risks, and trade-offs in national policy debates.[21]

To develop scenarios, teams of decision-makers, experts, and stakeholders generally meet at a 2- or 3-day workshop. The teams construct the scenarios by going through a process involving a series of steps. Specifically, they define a focal issue or decision, identify the main driving forces, write the scenario plots, flesh out the scenarios, look at the implications of the scenarios, choose leading indicators, and disseminate the scenarios. Generally, four or five scenarios are developed. Often one is the best-case scenario, which views the future optimistically. Another is the worst-case scenario, which views the future pessimistically. Other scenarios tend to be somewhere in between the two.[22–24]

A number of scenario analyses have been conducted to forecast the future of healthcare in the United States.[25–27]. An exemplar is the Robert Wood Johnson Foundation's *Health and Health Care in 2032*. Conducted by the Institute for Alternative Futures for the foundation, a national symposium of experts was held in 2012 to address the question: What do we want health and healthcare to be in the United States in 2032?

Four scenarios were developed to answer the question: Scenario 1—slow healthcare reform, leading to better health, it presents a conventional expectation assuming health, not healthcare becomes the main political issue; Scenario 2—health if you get it, it presents a growing desperation assuming severe budget cuts in Medicare and Medicaid and a growing number of uninsured; Scenario 3—big data, big health gains, it presents a high aspiration assuming health becomes a primary concern of government and the general population yielding cures for Alzheimer's disease and better cancer care; and Scenario 4—the establishment of a culture of health, it presents a high aspiration assuming leaders create environments to support and improve health.

These scenarios were then included in a matrix, and each was compared across multiple dimensions: U.S. economy, society and culture, government, definition of health, health threats, medical advances, healthcare delivery, health insurance coverage, health information technology, and national healthcare spending in 2032 as a percentage of GDP.

At the end of the symposium, the participants were asked to rank the four scenarios in terms of the likelihood of each occurring in the future. Scenario 1 was voted to be the most likely to occur, with Scenario 4 the least likely, and Scenario 2 and 3 fell between them. Last, areas of opportunity and recommendations to the nation were developed for each scenario.[28]

Strengths and weaknesses

Scenario analysis has the advantage of being a powerful tool to aid in decision-making. The scenarios can be beneficial for organizations and individuals to expand their views of the future. They can minimize surprises of what the future will bring. The scenarios also may improve communication through creating a common language for dealing with strategies to address the future.

However, scenario analysis has a number of disadvantages. The process of scenario development can be very time consuming. The scenarios are only as good as the individuals who develop them. They need to be developed by experts who have deep understandings and knowledge of the field under investigation. Last, the number of scenarios constructed may not include other more likely alternatives for the future.[29]

Conclusion

We will all live part of our lives in the future. Although it is very difficult to forecast and predict what lies ahead in the near and distant future, individuals, organizations, and governments must anticipate, prepare for, and attempt to shape the future. To move forward into the future, we will need roadmaps to guide us.

Futurists have provided us with some fundamental methods and tools needed to develop these maps. The maps will not be complete, but they will give us a rough idea of where we are going. Despite their limitations, we need to use them to better guide us and help us shape the future.[30–42]

The past cannot be changed, but the future is still within our power to change. Hopefully, we can change the future and make it better, healthier, safer, richer, and more rewarding for future generations. We owe them nothing less.

References

1. Asimov, I. 1965. Life in 1990. *Science Digest*, August, 58, 63.
2. Canton, J. 2015. *Future Smart: Managing the Game-Changing Trends that Will Transform Your World.* Boston, MA: Da Capo Press.
3. Gordan, A. 2008. *Future Savvy: Identifying Trends to Make Better Decisions, Manage Uncertainty, and Profit from Change.* New York, NY: American Management Association.

4. National Intelligence Council. 2004. *Mapping the Global Future: Report of the National Intelligence Council's 2020 Project*. Pittsburgh, PA: U.S. Government Printing Office. Available at: https://www.dni.gov/index.php/207-about/organization/national-intelligence-council/771-national-intelligence-council-global-trends-archive
5. United Nations, Department of Economic and Social Affairs, Population Division. 2015. *World Population Ageing Report*. New York, NY: United Nations. Available at www.un.org/en/development/desa/population/publications/pdf/ageing/WPA2015_Report.pdf
6. Thimbleby, H. 2013. Technology and the future of healthcare. *Journal of Public Health Research*, Dec. 1, 2(3), e28. Available at: https://archive.org/details/pubmed-PMC4147743
7. Garman, A. N., Johnson, T. J., Royer, T. C. 2011. *The Future of Healthcare: Global Trends Worth Watching*. Chicago, IL: Health Administration Press.
8. Coates, J. F., Jarratt, J. 1989. *What Futurists Believe*. Bethesda, MD: World Future Society.
9. Cornish, E. 2005. *Futuring: The Exploration of the Future*. Bethesda, MD: World Future Society.
10. Draper, N. R., Smith, H. 1998. *Applied Regression Analysis*. New York, NY: John Wiley and Sons.
11. Kahane, L. H. 2008. *Regression Basics*. Thousand Oaks, CA: Sage Publications.
12. Goldberg, M., Cho, H. A. 2010. *Introduction to Regression Analysis*. Billerica, MA: WIT Press.
13. Pampel, F. C. 2000. *Logistic Regression: A Primer*. Thousand Oaks, CA: Sage Publications.
14. Bagley, S. C., White, H., Golomb, B. A. 2001. Logistic regression in the medical literature: Standards for use and reporting, with particular attention to one medical domain. *Journal of Clinical Epidemiology*, 54(10) October, 979–985. Available at: https://www.researchgate.net
15. Linstone, H. A., Turoff, M. (Eds.). 1975. *The Delphi Method: Techniques and Applications*. Reading, MA: Addison-Wesley.
16. Adler, M., Ziglio, E. (Eds.). 1996. *Gazing into the Oracle: The Delphi Method and Its Application to Social Policy and Public Health*. Bristol, PA: Jessica Kingsley Publishers.
17. Keeney, S., Hasson, F., McKenna, H. 2011. *The Delphi Technique in Nursing and Health Research*. New York, NY: Wiley-Blackwell.
18. American Hospital Association. 2018. *The 2018 AHA Environmental Scan: Trends that Are Shaping Health Care*. Chicago, IL: American Hospital Association. Available at: https://www.aha.org/2018-environmental-scan
19. Fine, L. G. 2010. *The SWOT Analysis: Using Your Strength to Overcome Weaknesses, Using Opportunities to Overcome Threat*. North Charleston, SC: Creatspace.
20. Gray, C. S. et al. 2016. eHealth advances in support of people with complex care needs: Case examples from Canada, Scotland, and the U.S. *Healthcare Quarterly*, 19(2), July, 29–37. Available at: https://www.researchgate.net
21. Chermack, T. J. 2011. *Scenario Planning in Organizations: How to Create, Use, and Assess Scenarios*. San Francisco, CA: Berrett-Koehler Press.
22. Maack, J. N. 2001. Scenario Analysis: A Tool for Task Managers. In: *Social Analysis: Selected Tools and Techniques*. R. A. Krueger et al. Social Development Papers, No. 36. Washington, DC: The World Bank, 62–87. Available at: http://citeseerx.ist.psu.edu/viewdoc/download?doi=10.1.1.607.4701&rep=rep1&type=pdf
23. Schoemaker, P. J. H. 1993. Multiple scenario development: Its conceptual and behavioral foundation. *Strategic Management Journal*, 14(3) March, 193–213. Available at: https://www.researchgate.net
24. Werner, R. R. 2010. *Designing Strategy: The Art of Scenario Analysis*. Chagrin Falls, OH: Windjammer Adventure Publishing.
25. Bezold, C. 1994. Scenarios for 21st-century health care in the United States of America: Perspectives on time and change. *World Health Statistics Quarterly*, 47(3–4), 126–139.
26. Facility Guidelines Institute. 2015. *The Future of Health Care as Predicted Using Scenario Planning: A Summary*. Chicago, IL: American Society for Healthcare Engineering of the

American Hospital Association. Available at: https://www.fgiguidelines.org/wp-content/uploads/2015/07/FGI
27. Institute for the Future. 2009. *Healthcare 2020 Perspectives*. Palo Alto, CA: Institute for the Future. Available at: http://www.iftf.org
28. Institute for Alternative Futures. 2012. *Health and Health Care in 2032: Report from the Robert Wood Johnson Foundation Futures Symposium, June 20–21, 2012, Alexandria, VA*. Alexandria, VA: Institute for Alternative Futures. Available at: https://altfutures.org/pubs/RWJF/IAF-HealthandHealthCare2032.pdf
29. Mietzner, D., Reger, G. 2005. Advantages and disadvantages of scenario approaches for strategic foresight. *International Journal of Technology Intelligence and Planning*, 1(2), 220–239. Available at SSRN: https://ssrn.com/abstract=1736110
30. Bari, A., Chaouchi, M., Jung, T. 2017. *Predictive Analytics for Dummies*. Hoboken, NJ: John Wiley and Sons.
31. "By the Year 2050...". 2011. In the future. *Lapham's Quarterly*, 4(4) Fall, 10–11.
32. Damberg, C. L. et al. 2014. *Measuring Success in Health Care Value-Based Purchasing Programs: Findings from an Environmental Scan, Literature Review, and Expert Panel Discussions. Research Report*. Santa Monica, CA: RAND Corporation. Available at: http://www.rand.org/pubs/research_reports/RR306z1.html
33. Gallant, M., Szaro, B. 2016. *Futuring Paper—Health Sciences and Public Health*. Albany, NY: University of Albany, State University of New York. Available at: https:// www.albany.edu/strategicplan/
34. Graham, P., Evitts, T., Thomas-MacLean, R. 2008. Environmental scans: How useful are they for primary care research? *Canadian Family Physicians*, 54(7), July, 1022–1023. Available at: https://www.cfp.ca/content/54/7/1022.short
35. Institute of Medicine. 2003. *The Future of the Public's Health in the 21st Century*. Washington, DC: National Academies Press.
36. Kuhn, M., Johnson, K. 2016. *Applied Predictive Modeling*. New York, NY: Springer Science-Business Media.
37. Lempert, R. J., Popper, S. W., Bankes, S. C. 2003. *Shaping the Next One Hundred Years: New Methods for Quantitative, Long-Term Policy Analysis*. Santa Monica, CA: RAND Corporation. Available at: https://www.rand.org
38. Lesca, N. (Ed.). 2013. *Environmental Scanning and Sustainable Development*. New York, NY: John Wiley and Sons.
39. National Academies of Sciences, Engineering, and Medicine. 2016. *Exploring Data and Metrics of Value at the Intersection of Health Care and Transportation: Proceedings of a Workshop*. Washington, DC: National Academies Press.
40. Rose, P. 2016. *The Future Belongs to Those Who Dare: Choosing Your Life through Strategic Futuring*. Yorba Linda, CA: Genysys Group.
41. Schimpff, S. C. 2012. *The Future of Health-Care Delivery: Why It Must Change and How It Will Affect You*. Dulles, VA: Potomac Books.
42. Schwartz, P. 1996. *The Art of the Long View: Planning for the Future in an Uncertain World*. New York, NY: Currency Doubleday.

Chapter 7

Conclusion

Ross M. Mullner and Edward M. Rafalski

CONTENTS

As structured today, the healthcare system in the United States faces a number of problems and paradoxes. First, the United States spends an inordinate amount of money on healthcare delivery, i.e., 18% of gross domestic product, but relatively little on evaluating the efficacy and efficiency of delivering that care and its resulting outcomes. The United States spends an estimated 5.6% of its total health expenditures on biomedical research, although less than 0.1% is allocated to health services research.[1] Healthcare organizations, providers specifically, may spend up to 0.2% of overall net revenues on health services or outcomes research. By contrast, information technology represents 4.4% of net revenues.[2] Two areas where additional resources have been allocated include clinical quality and, for those healthcare systems embracing risk contracting, population health analytics.

In the former case, advancements in value-based purchasing, where providers are rewarded for quality clinical outcomes and publically reported measures, as reported by the Centers for Medicare and Medicaid Services, have enticed health systems to allocate more resources to analyze financial cost/benefit and clinical outcomes performance. However, the benefits of reducing hospital re-admissions, a publically reported measure, for example, are still far outweighed by the net revenue gained from the re-admissions. In other words, the penalties are not sufficient. So, while systems may analyze re-admission prevention, the financial incentive still resides in the hospital admission, where running more tests and performing more procedures in a fee-for-service reimbursement model generate more revenue for the health system and the physicians ordering the tests and performing the procedures. This financial perversion leads to systems investing more in financial analysis as opposed to outcomes research.

In the latter case, for those systems embracing population health as they move down the road to assuming more financial risk, particularly those providers who are pursuing a provider-sponsored health insurance offering, additional resources are being added to outcomes research. Arguably, the merging of health insurance companies and healthcare providers may be leading to the investment in health outcomes research, although we are early in that market evolution.

Second, much of the healthcare provided has not been subjected to rigorous clinical trial, so most of the time healthcare providers do not know what works and what does not. In those instances where pharmacological providers are interested in testing new interventions, clinical trials are funded to prove that innovations in drug therapy are efficacious. This is more likely the case in academic medical centers and less so in community-based provider settings, of which there are significantly more in the United States. Further, clinical trials are time consuming and costly.

Third, secondary data is available but not used for significant outcomes research. There are billions of patient records, but they are not rigorously analyzed. Recent investments and mergers in computer technology purveyors, such as with IBM Watson/Truven Analytics and Optum/Healthcare Advisory Board, have led to some initial work, but arguably there are many more analytical opportunities to be leveraged. Machine learning, natural language processing, and clinical algorithms have evolved to a point where social capital can be leveraged to transform the healthcare industry through analytics. Social capital may be defined as comprising the networks of relationships among people who live and work in a particular society, enabling that society to function effectively. Social capital exists where people have an advantage because of their location in social structure.[3] The advance of technology and healthcare industry orientation are enabling the patient/consumer to connect with the delivery system in a manner that was not possible a decade or so ago. The ability to leverage large data sets, both clinical and consumer, allows for the healthcare analyst to observe patterns of interaction and derive insights that can be applied to improve health outcomes. Arguably, these observed interactions between the healthcare system and consumer enable the creation of social health capital. If we can learn what motivates a consumer to engage in his or her health, this will thereby lead to a more productive and healthy life and will benefit society as a whole. More effective consumer engagement makes the healthcare system more effective because we are not just relying on the primary care provider to drive health improvement in a brief annual encounter, year over year; we are relying on multiple data input nodes that enable trending analysis daily, weekly, and monthly. Health improvement occurs in increments, and by definition those increments must be observed more frequently than once per year.

Fourth, the cost of investing in computer technology and calculations has declined to the point where an individual at his or her home can analyze large data sets. We are entering an age where the computing power is relatively low cost, enabling new breakthroughs in healthcare analytics. If only we could harness the intellectual prowess of computer hackers to spend time on improving society and creating social health capital. The analysis of data, especially large disparate data sets, is now possible. We are at an inflection point in the evolution of the healthcare system, where new questions to problems can be answered.

The future of healthcare analytics requires that we develop a fundamental understanding of the health of populations and the determinants of health, both clinical and social. Clinical disease will always exist, although the leading causes of death will shift over time. For example, diabetes is the leading cause of death in Mexico, responsible for 14.7% of the deaths in that country. The percentage of the population that has died of this disease has tripled since 1990, and it is predicted that half of the population will suffer from the disease by 2050.[4] The underlying cause of the increase in the death rate has less to do with clinical vectors but everything to do with changes in diet that began in the 1970s. Understanding aspects of rising clinical risk can lead to fundamental learning opportunities to preventing the onset of chronic disease.

The ability to leverage complex data sets, both structured and unstructured, can enable the healthcare analyst to harness the power of computing to find answers to complex problems. As recently as 20 years ago, the healthcare analyst would take the better part of a week to analyze a small data set, such as inpatient hospital physician length of stay, written with fairly straightforward code that led to the creation of a print file that would be transformed to a database file that could be analyzed using a spreadsheet program. Now, that calculation can be done in a few minutes. Complex health risk equations are solved in nanoseconds.

The evolution of bioinformatics as a discipline has led to a framework, knowledge management, which is the academic discipline that studies and effects the transformation of data into actionable information. This has enabled the transition from the creation of data to the creation of actionable information. The evolution of geospatial analytics adds to the framework, transforming data from columns and rows to a third plane, space. We can now analyze outcomes in visual maps, which enable the analyst to draw conclusions that may not have been as readily evident, such as the disparity in access to screening technology by race, which leads to disparity in mortality caused by structural access problems.[5,6]

Being able to peer into the future using historical analysis is not a new concept. Yet, we are now able to model future outcomes based on historical data and predict various scenarios. Among other models, game theory has a place in healthcare, creating win-win scenarios among disparate organizations that are coming together in the disruption of the industry.

The skills needed to perform the analytics necessary to draw inferences from multiple data nodes are varied. No one skill necessarily dominates the analytical frontier. The healthcare analyst becomes a combination of statistician, database architect, bio-informaticist, cartographer, epidemiologist, clinician, and administrator. Academic programs preparing the future analyst arguably need to create curricula that combine elements of each of the aforementioned disciplines. The most valued analyst will be the one who can translate across multiple disciplines to provide insights that will advance the work of building systems of health and to create ecosystems that create social health capital.

References

1. Krumholz, H. 2008. Outcomes research generating evidence for best practice and policies. *Circulation*, 118, 309–318.
2. Gartner. Available at: https://www.gartner.com/document/3832566?ref=cust_reco_sdemail
3. Burt, S. R., Ronchi, D. 2006. Teaching executives to see social capital: Results from a field experiment. *Social Science Research*, 36, 1156–1183.
4. Biomedical Engineering. *Diabetes: Leading Cause of Death in Mexico.* Available at: https://www.bu.edu/globalhealthtechnologies/2017/04/18/diabetes-leading-cause-of-death-in-mexico/
5. Rauscher, G. et al. 2012. Disparities in screening mammography services by race/ethnicity and health insurance. *Journal of Women's Health*, 21(2), 154–160.
6. Ansell D. et al. A community effort to reduce the black/white breast cancer mortality disparity in Chicago. *Cancer Causes Control.* 20, 1681–1688.

Index

For Product Safety Concerns and Information please contact our EU representative GPSR@taylorandfrancis.com Taylor & Francis Verlag GmbH, Kaufingerstraße 24, 80331 München, Germany

Batch number: 10726412

Printed by Printforce, the Netherlands